RADIANT WELLNESS

A Transformative Journey to Vitality
and Longevity through Clean Living, Emotional
Renewal, and Energetic Healing

DENISE CAHILL, CNC

Copyright © 2025 Denise Cahill

All rights reserved.

No portion of this book may be reproduced in any form without written permission from the publisher or author, except as permitted by U.S. copyright law.

This publication is designed to provide accurate and authoritative information in regard to the subject matter covered. It is sold with the understanding that neither the author nor the publisher is engaged in rendering legal, medical, psychiatric or other professional services. While the publisher and author have used their best efforts in preparing this book, they make no representations or warranties with respect to the accuracy or completeness of the contents of this book and specifically disclaim any implied warranties of merchantability or fitness for a particular purpose. No warranty may be created or extended by sales representatives or written sales materials. The advice and strategies contained herein may not be suitable for your situation. You should consult with a professional when appropriate. Neither the publisher nor the author shall be liable for any loss of profit or any other commercial damages, including but not limited to special, incidental, consequential, personal, or other damages.

Modern Wellness Publishing

1st printing 2025

ISBN: 979-8-9987500-3-8

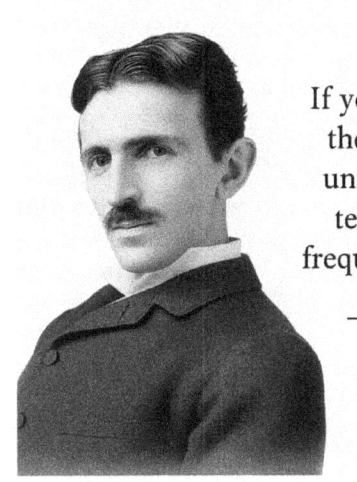

If you want to know the secrets of the universe, think in terms of energy, frequency & vibration.

– Nikola Tesla

Product and Brand Disclosure

Throughout this book, I mention certain products, devices, and brands that I personally use, know of, or recommend for educational purposes. These references are provided solely as examples to support your wellness journey. I have no financial affiliation with any of the companies mentioned, nor do I receive compensation, commissions, or incentives for including these recommendations.

Author Affiliation Disclosure

SoulScans is a wellness service I personally created and offer through my practice. References to SoulScans are included to help readers explore energy-based wellness tools and not intended as endorsements or paid advertisements.

Contents

Preface	1
Introduction to Holistic Health	3
PART ONE: ENERGY AND THE VIBRANT BODY	9
1. Food for Thought	15
2. Removing Toxins in Our Diet	17
3. Read the Labels!	49
4. Limiting Toxins from Our Homes	53
5. EMFs & Radiation	61
6. Gut Health	65
7. Food Allergies vs. Food Sensitivities	85
8. The Truth About Supplements	89
9. Acidic vs. Alkaline Foods	95
10. The Glycemic Index	99
11. High Vibrational Foods	103
12. Transitioning to a Healthy Diet	109
13. #1 Recipe for Health Smoothies!	111
14. Dietary Guidelines	117
15. Meat. To Eat or Not to Eat?	121

16.	Hydration for Vitality	129
17.	Daily Detox	133
18.	Exercise Your Way to Radiance	141
19.	Sleep Yourself Well	147
20.	Holistic Dental Health & Biological Dentistry	155
PART TWO: THE MIND-BODY CONNECTION		159
21.	The Emotional Blueprint of Disease	165
22.	Understanding Chronic Stress	171
23.	Emotional Mastery	179
24.	Cultivating Happiness & Joy	187
25.	Consciousness & Mindset	207
26.	Emotional Healing Through Self-Reflection	227
27.	Meditation: The Science of Stillness	235
PART THREE: BIOFREQUENCY FOR VIBRANT HEALTH		239
28.	Bioenergetic Testing	241
29.	Rife Machines	247
30.	Acupuncture	251
31.	Cold Laser Therapy	255
32.	Sound Therapy	261
33.	Color Therapy	271
34.	Scalar Energy	279
35.	The Biomat	281
36.	Wearable Frequency Patches	285
37.	PEMF	291
38.	BioCharger NG	297

Preface

I've always been fascinated by what lies beneath the surface and the mysteries of the body, mind, and universe that science can't quite explain. I believe it's safe to say that I am a wellness geek and a truth-seeker. I do my research, and if something doesn't feel right, it generally isn't.

I came to where I am in my holistic health journey not overnight but over a lifelong stance of paying attention. As a child, I questioned everything and was in awe of anything that seemed mystic or mysterious. At the age of 10, I was intrigued by the prophecies of Nostradamus. At 12, I questioned several aspects of my religion. In my early 20s, everything I believed about healing was shaken when my mother passed away from cancer shortly after chemotherapy. Watching her fade despite doing "everything right" lit a fire in me to determine and understand what true healing really means. That moment launched me down a lifelong rabbit hole—one that began with *The Creature from Jekyll Island* and hasn't stopped expanding since. Each page, each documentary, each conversation peeled back another layer of illusion, revealing how much more there is to health, energy, and consciousness than we're ever taught. My last corporate job in the biomedical field taught me that our healthcare system was often controlled by profits rather than our best interests.

Year after year, in my spare time and on vacations, I gravitated toward reading health and self-help books instead of the newest and best-selling fiction novels. Eventually, I walked away from the corporate world to pursue something that truly fed my soul. I formally studied nutrition and naturopathy, and from that moment on, there was no looking back.

When I opened my first wellness center, my world transformed. I found myself surrounded by intuitive healers, reiki masters, shamans, and teachers of ancient wisdom—all of which I knew very little about. It felt as if the universe had placed me exactly where I needed to be—in the heart of a community that spoke the language my soul had been yearning for.

My motivation for writing Radiant Wellness is to empower my clients and readers with knowledge of various topics that may improve their health utilizing a holistic approach that is often not discussed within the conventional medical system. The combination of Western medicine and holistic healing therapies can be the perfect complement to each other to speed up the healing process if used correctly.

Whether you're just beginning your holistic journey or have been walking this path for years, this book was written for you—the seeker, the skeptic, the soul hungry for radiant wellness.

Our goal should not be to live forever but, while living, to have the best health and well-being possible so that we can live a life free of pain, trauma, stress, dis-ease, and emotional turmoil to enjoy a sacred life without all the distractions keeping us from maintaining a deeper connection to our true selves. My hope is that you will find valuable information within the pages of this book to guide you on a beautiful path of existence.

Introduction to Holistic Health

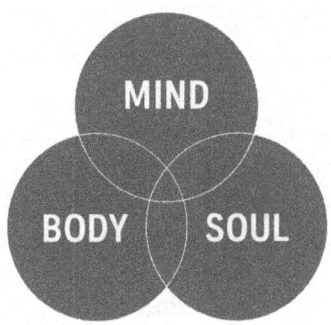

As an introduction to holistic health, we will discuss the basic principles and how it fits into allopathic or mainstream medicine as well as the various types of doctors, and their common methodologies.

Understanding Holistic Health: Nurturing the Whole Person

Holistic health is an approach to well-being that views a person as an integrated whole—body, mind, emotions, and spirit—rather than a collection of separate symptoms or organs. Instead of focusing solely on relieving discomfort, holistic health seeks to uncover the root causes of imbalance, supporting the body's innate ability to heal. The goal is not merely the absence of disease, but a vibrant state of vitality and resilience.

The core Principles of Holistic Health include:

- **The Whole-Person Perspective.** Health is a dynamic interaction between physical, emotional, mental, spiritual, social, and environmental factors. Each aspect influences the others: emotional stress can create physical tension; nutrient deficiencies can cloud mental focus; spiritual stagnation can lower motivation and vitality.

- **Prevention and Root-Cause Healing.** Rather than waiting for illness to appear, holistic care emphasizes lifestyle choices, early detection of imbalances, and strengthening the body's natural defenses. It asks *why* symptoms arise and works to correct underlying causes such as poor nutrition, chronic stress, or environmental toxins.

- **The Body's Innate Healing Wisdom.** The human organism is designed for self-repair—cells regenerate, wounds close, and immune defenses activate. Holistic care enhances these natural mechanisms with supportive practices instead of suppressing them with quick fixes.

- **Individualization.** No two people share the same genetic, emotional, or environmental profile. Holistic practitioners tailor interventions, nutrition plans, herbal protocols, and movement routines, to the unique needs of each individual.

- **Mind-Body-Spirit Connection.** Thoughts, emotions, and spiritual beliefs influence physical health through neurochemical and hormonal pathways. Practices such as meditation, gratitude, and mindful movement help harmonize these subtle yet powerful forces.

The key modalities and practices include:

- **Nutrition and Clean Eating.** Food is both fuel and information. A colorful, whole-food diet rich in antioxidants, fiber, and phytonutrients provides the building blocks for cellular repair and vibrant energy. Holistic nutrition considers food's energetic properties—fresh, living foods are thought to convey higher "life force," while ultra-processed foods diminish vitality.

- **Movement and Physical Alignment.** Exercise is not only for muscles; it benefits the heart, lymphatic system, brain chemistry, and emotional balance. Practices like yoga, tai chi, Pilates, and mindful walking integrate breath, posture, and awareness.

- **Energy Medicine and Subtle Therapies.** Modalities such as energy healing and biofrequency treatments aim to balance the body's subtle energy fields and will be covered in Part Three. While research continues to explore their mechanisms, many people report improved health, profound relaxation, pain relief, and emotional release.

- **Mind-Body Practices.** Meditation, breathwork, guided imagery, and journaling reduce stress hormones, improve focus, and create inner peace. Regular self-reflection, referred to as soul diving or shadow work, helps process emotions and release patterns that no longer serve us.

- **Detoxification and Environmental Awareness.** Holistic health recognizes the impact of environmental toxins, heavy metals, and chronic inflammation. Supportive strategies may include liver-friendly foods, hydration, infrared sauna, and mindful use of household products.

- **Spiritual Connection and Purpose.** Whether through prayer, nature immersion, or acts of service, cultivating a sense of meaning strengthens emotional resilience and can positively influence physical health.

The core science behind holistic principles are as follows:

- **Systems Biology: The Body as an Ecosystem.** The human organism operates as a complex network of cells, organs, microbes, and hormones that communicate through chemical and electrical signals. Systems biology research shows that a disturbance in one part (e.g., chronic stress elevating cortisol) can cascade into others, affecting immune function, metabolism, and mood.

- **Root-Cause Medicine.** Conditions like Type 2 diabetes, hypertension, and many autoimmune diseases often stem from lifestyle and environmental triggers. Functional medicine and integrative healthcare focus on correcting dietary imbalances, nutrient deficiencies, and chronic inflammation, rather than only controlling symptoms with medication.

- **The Mind–Body Connection.** Neuroscience demonstrates that mental states shape physiology: stress activates the hypothalamic–pituitary–adrenal (HPA) axis, influencing immune cells and gut microbiota. Practices like meditation and breathwork measurably lower blood pressure, modulate gene expression, and improve heart-rate variability.

- **Epigenetics and Gene Expression.** Genes are not destiny. Research shows that nutrition, stress, and physical activity can turn genes "on" or "off," affecting disease risk and longevity. This epigenetic insight underscores how lifestyle choices are potent therapeutic tools.

Collaboration with Healthcare Providers

Holistic health complements conventional care in a more complete way. Integrative medicine centers and hospital-based lifestyle clinics use nutritionists, physicians, and mind-body specialists to develop individualized plans. Major U.S. centers, such as the Cleveland Clinic, Mayo Clinic, and MD Anderson Cancer Center, operate integrative medicine departments. Medical schools increasingly teach lifestyle and mind-body topics. This collaborative model ensures that evidence-based natural therapies enhance, rather than replace, essential medical treatments. When shopping for a physician, it is helpful to know the specifics of each type of practice and what values you are seeking. Modern health care includes several categories of licensed doctors. Knowing how each is educated and how they practice can help you choose the care, or combination of care, that fits your needs.

- **Medical Doctor (MD)**. MDs are physicians trained in allopathic (conventional Western) medicine. They are licensed to diagnose disease, prescribe medications, perform surgery, and practice in every medical specialty (from pediatrics and family medicine to cardiology and neurosurgery). Their education and training includes: 4 years of undergraduate study (usually science-focused), 4 years of medical school with rigorous biomedical and clinical sciences, 3–7+ years of residency, plus optional fellowship training, National board exams (USMLE in the United States) and state licensure. Their philosophy and scope emphasize pharmaceuticals, surgery, and technology. MD-programs in the U.S., generally do *not* devote a lot of time or resources to nutrition or preventative medicine. This category is the most common to date and is covered by most medical insurance companies.

- **Doctor of Osteopathic Medicine (DO)**. DOs are fully licensed physicians with the same prescribing and surgical rights as MDs. They practice in all specialties, from primary care to surgery. Their education and training are Similar academic pathway: 4-year undergraduate degree, 4-year osteopathic medical school, and residency/fellowship. They must pass the COMLEX licensing exam (and often the USMLE as well). Their distinctive features include whole-person philosophy: DO training includes the belief that structure and function of the body are interrelated and that the body has an innate ability to heal itself. The use of Osteopathic Manipulative Treatment (OMT) offers hands-on techniques to diagnose, treat, and help prevent conditions by improving musculoskeletal alignment, circulation, and nervous system function. Their emphasis is on primary care and preventive medicine, though many specialize in surgery, cardiology, or other advanced fields.

- **Naturopathic Doctor (ND or NMD).** The titles ND and NMD are equivalent; some U.S. states use NMD—"Naturopathic Medical Doctor"—to emphasize clinical training. Naturopathic doctors, also referred to as licensed naturopathic doctors, are trained in natural and integrative medicine. They focus on supporting the body's inherent healing capacity through nutrition, lifestyle, herbal medicine, homeopathy, physical medicine, and mind–body techniques. In some licensed states, they may prescribe certain medications, order labs and imaging, and perform minor procedures. Their education and training include a 4-year undergraduate degree with a science prerequisite, a 4-year accredited naturopathic medical program including basic sciences (anatomy, physiology, biochemistry) and natural therapeutics, national board exams (NPLEX) plus state licensing where regulation exists. Their practice consists of a root-cause, patient-centered approach emphasizing prevention and lifestyle medicine. They may use botanical medicine, nutritional therapy, hydrotherapy, acupuncture, and energy-based modalities alongside conventional diagnostics. Regulation varies by region: in licensed states such as Arizona, Washington, and Oregon, NDs/NMDs function as primary care physicians; elsewhere they may serve as wellness consultants. Most insurance providers do not cover this type of alternative medicine but may vary by state. Check with your coverage beforehand and plan ahead for any out-of-pocket expenses.

Many patients find the best results by combining these strengths and seeing an MD or DO for acute illness, advanced imaging, and necessary prescriptions, and working with an NMD/ND for nutritional optimization, lifestyle transformation, and natural therapies. However, there is one more doctor that must be included for optimal health.

- **YOU.** You are your best doctor. Why? Because no one spends more time inside your body than you. You're the first to notice subtle shifts such as changes in mood, energy, digestion, or sleep that rarely appear on lab tests. Doctors, even the most caring, typically see you for 15 minutes during your appointment. They rely on vitals, lab numbers, and your complaints and symptoms. While a doctor can guide and interpret, the deepest knowledge of how food, lifestyle, stress, and environment affect you is something only you can fully observe. If you are not willing or able to prepare healthy meals or deal with your stress, seek out help from a qualified professional.

In addition, it is important to be proactive with your own research, prescriptions, and care plans. It is true that modern medicine saves lives, but it is also complex and profit driven. For example, every (and I do mean *every*) prescription and over-the-counter drug, has side effects and interactions that carry risks. Do a quick internet search before starting any new treatment. This goes for herbal supplements, tinctures and nutritional supplements as well. Everyone is different. Between genetics, gut microbiome, stress levels, and diet, each person may metabolize a substance differently. In other words, a drug or supplement may be an excellent solution for one person or the "average patient" in trials or studies, but that person may not be *you*. By reading the prescribing information, checking reliable databases (e.g., NIH, MedlinePlus, PubMed), and asking precise questions, you become an informed partner in your own care. This isn't distrust; it's due diligence—the same care you'd take when signing a financial contract or making a major purchase.

PART ONE: ENERGY AND THE VIBRANT BODY

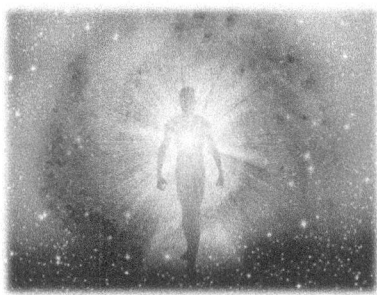

The human body comprises both the physical body and the light body. The physical body includes the mechanical, physical, bioelectrical, and biochemical functions from organs to our trillions of cells. Science provides us with ongoing information of the energetic nature of the body's inner workings. To this day, scientists are still studying the energetic nature within the nucleus of the atom and the orbiting electrons. Scientific research suggests that there is a holographic nature to biology. A hologram is defined as a three-dimensional image formed by the interference of light beams from a laser or other coherent light source. The existence of this subtle body is not only becoming verified, but it may answer the question of what intelligent force instructs our DNA to build our bodies properly. Further research suggests that our DNA acts as an antenna to read and convert subtle energetic resonance from a larger, collective morphic field related to the human body. These studies also suggest that our lifestyles, emotional states and intentions are powerful enough to alter our chromosomes, as in the study of epigenetics.

Understanding the Energy-Frequency-Vibration Concept. Energy can be a complicated subject especially regarding how all of this equates to our health. Let's start by breaking down each of the three components of energy, frequency and vibration, and how they flow together.

Energy. In a nutshell, everything in existence (stars, oceans, forests, human bodies, plants, animals, and even inanimate objects) is made of energy. Atoms are not solid particles but dynamic clouds of subatomic activity. This ceaseless motion creates subtle fields of energy that influence and are influenced by everything around them. Whether we call it chi, prana, or life force, this energy animates us and forms the invisible architecture of health.

Energy is the foundation of all existence. From the electricity that powers a heartbeat to the chemical energy stored in food, every life process depends on it. Human beings are bioelectrical organisms:

The heart generates a magnetic field measurable several feet away.

Neurons fire electrical impulses that create recognizable brainwave patterns.

Every cell communicates through tiny electromagnetic signals.

When this energy flows freely, we feel vital. When it is blocked or incoherent, we may experience fatigue, illness, or emotional distress.

Frequency. If energy is motion, frequency is the speed of that motion—measured in hertz (cycles per second). Examples include:

Brain Waves: Delta (0.5–4 Hz) for deep sleep, Alpha (8–12 Hz) for calm focus, Gamma (~40 Hz) for insight.

Heart Rhythms: Coherent heart-rate variability is linked to emotional resilience and reduced stress.

Musical notes and colors each have distinct frequencies.

Many holistic traditions teach that each cell, organ, and even thought has a "signature frequency." While modern science confirms that tissues exhibit electromagnetic properties, the idea that an overall "personal frequency" can be expressed in a single hertz number remains a metaphor rather than a measurable quantity.

Vibration. Where frequency is a numerical rate, vibration is the texture and quality of the movement.

We feel vibration when a singing bowl hums or when the body tingles during meditation.

Emotions influence vibration: gratitude and joy create coherent heart and brain patterns, while fear and anger create chaotic ones.

Though not a literal "buzz" of thousands of hertz, these vibrational qualities can dramatically shape mental and physical well-being.

Food and Frequency. Real food is condensed sunlight and earth energy. It nourishes not only chemically but vibrationally. Scientists use advanced instruments to analyze foods' molecular motion and electromagnetic signatures:

- Near-Infrared (NIR) Spectroscopy detects sugars, proteins, and moisture by reading how molecules absorb light frequencies.

- Dielectric or Impedance Analysis measures how food responds to alternating electrical fields to gauge freshness and ripeness.

- Nuclear Magnetic Resonance (NMR) Spectroscopy reads the resonant behavior of atoms to reveal composition.

These tools measure genuine electromagnetic properties, but no instrument confirms a spiritual "frequency in hertz" that makes food high or low-vibration. Nevertheless, fresh, whole, minimally processed foods do support vitality—aligning with both science and traditional wisdom about "living foods."

A Spiritual View of High Frequency Living (aka High Consciousness Living). Many traditions speak of the spiritual energy of people we might call high-frequency beings. Jesus of Nazareth radiated unconditional love and forgiveness, qualities described in mystical Christianity as "Christ Consciousness." Mahatma Gandhi lived ahimsa, or non-violence, mobilizing entire nations through moral clarity and peace. Siddhartha Gautama (the Buddha) embodied a very high spiritual frequency—meaning a consciousness of profound love, peace, and enlightenment.

The deeper truth is metaphorical: their lives demonstrated states of coherence, compassion, and love so profound that people felt uplifted simply in their presence. These qualities, while not quantifiable in hertz, do correspond to measurable physiological benefits, calm nervous systems, lowered stress hormones, and stronger immunity. Modern books sometimes claim that such figures vibrated at 700–1000 Hz, a concept inspired partly by David R. Hawkins' *Map of Consciousness*. These measurements were obtained through applied kinesiology or muscle testing. Hawkins then assigned numbers from 1 to 1,000 to represent these states. Through this method, he also revealed a universal calibration of the level of consciousness of emotions. For example, shame = 20, guilt = 30, fear = 100, courage = 200, love = 500, enlightenment = 700–1,000. He often referred to these numbers as frequencies or vibrations, but they are not physical hertz.

Energy, frequency, and vibration are not just buzzwords or rhetoric. They are the very foundation of life. Science can measure certain electromagnetic rhythms of the brain, heart, and food. Spiritual traditions remind us that love, service, and inner peace raise the frequency of our consciousness in ways that instruments may never capture. Understanding both aspects allows us to live more fully: to eat foods rich in natural vitality, to calm and focus the mind, to cultivate love and compassion, and to participate in the great symphony of life as conscious co-creators. Simply stated, low-vibrational states are intended to keep us sick, unnourished, stressed, and emotionally void, blocking our connection to our life force energy, intuition, creativity, and our higher self. Just by raising our vibrational energy, we can create a life of radiance and vitality.

Universal Laws. Universal laws are *natural laws*. Meaning these laws are fundamental principles governing the universe. They are innate and unchanging, operating across all situations, and not created by humans. In other words, they have not been created by any specific society or authority and are considered inherent to the universe. They are often associated with concepts such as physics and the natural order of things, including the law of gravity. They can be observed in various fields, including law, ethics, science, and philosophy.

These laws pertain to energy and vibration and how they impact our lives. The Law of Vibration states that everything vibrates, including thoughts and emotions. The Law of Resonance states that vibrations with similar frequencies attract and amplify each other. The Law of Mentalism states that the universe is mental and that our thoughts and beliefs shape the world around us.

Through these principles, we believe that with every thought, feeling, word, or action we create, our life force flows on an electromagnetic energy current similar to how radio and television waves pass through the atmosphere. Our energy current vibrates with the frequency of vibration we charge it with, depending on the mood and expressions we emit within every moment. As our current of energy travels throughout the universe, it accumulates other energy vibrating at the same frequency. Like magnets, we attract similar energies to those we transmit back into our lives. Consequently, raising our vibration will allow us to attract positive experiences and manifest incredible things.

Just as with the foods we eat to raise our vibration, we can increase our vibrational energy with the actions, thoughts, and words we choose to use. This practice affects our lives personally and can raise the vibration of the entire planet as we become a powerful antenna of universal light, one thought or action at a time. It's a complex concept to grasp, yet it is confirmed throughout the scientific world through the science of quantum entanglement.

The Water Experiment. Performed in 1999, Dr. Masaru Emoto set out to demonstrate that words, thoughts, and emotions carry vibrational energy. He conducted a series of experiments to test the effects of words, thoughts, and emotions on water. When he began his experiments, he wanted to test his hypothesis that water could react to both positive and negative thoughts and words. He wrote or spoke words such as love, happiness, hope, and I love you into pure water. He also used words like evil, I hate you, and you make me sick. After doing this, he froze the water and used a specialized microscope to observe the crystalline structures that formed. The water with the positive, high-vibrational words created beautifully structured patterns. The ugly, low-vibrational words could not form any pattern at all. In fact, they looked like disturbing, distorted blobs.

He continued experimenting and discovered that vibrational frequency also played a role, comparing the effects of loud, heavy metal music with those of soft, soothing melodies containing positive and uplifting messages. This leads us to the powerful conclusion that the things to which we expose ourselves—whether words, thoughts, or sounds—have immense implications for our health and well-being.

Section One Overview. In this section, we will journey into all things physical to inspire vibrant health and wellness. Our bodies are not merely vessels, but a sacred instrument of expression, vitality, and resonance.

We will cover how high-vibrational foods, clean eating, and mindful nourishment serve as fuel not just for growth, but for transformation and sustainable health. Detoxification is explored as releasing what no longer serves, clearing the way for clarity, energy, and resilience deep within. Movement is celebrated not merely as calorie burn, but as purposeful, joyous activation of every cell, reconnecting us with strength and resilience for life.

Sleep is honored not as downtime, but as a powerful reset, our body's essential time to recharge, balance hormones, support immunity, and integrate everything we've eaten, done, thought, and felt. Optimal rest allows repair, growth, and deeper connection to your inner wisdom.

Hydration carries us, quite literally. Clean and intentional fluid intake supports every system: nutrient transport, detox, energy, cognitive clarity, mood, and overall flow. Hydration elevated beyond mere thirst becomes part of the energetic language that the body speaks.

Together, by aligning nutrition, meaningful movement, restorative sleep, and energetic awareness, we will learn to cultivate a body that is inherently balanced, powerful, and in harmony with our highest potential, thriving not just today, but for lifelong vitality.

Chapter 1
Food for Thought

The food we consume can either heal or harm us. As the saying goes, *"garbage in, garbage out."* When we feed the body with clean, living nutrients, we fuel our cells with vitality and energy. When we feed it with artificial, processed foods filled with chemicals, preservatives, and toxins, we drain that vitality and create imbalance.

In the modern world, much of our food has become far removed from its natural state. Industrialization and mass production have altered the way food is grown, processed, and prepared. The result? Foods that look appealing but are depleted of life force, enzymes, and nutrients.

The human body is an extraordinary, self-healing organism that depends on what we put into it. Every bite we take either contributes to health or to disease. Choosing clean, whole foods allows our body to function in harmony with nature and the universe, maintaining higher energy and vibrational frequency.

Unfortunately, the convenience-driven food industry has replaced much of what was once nourishing with highly processed, refined, and chemical-laden alternatives. These substances may satisfy taste buds but leave the body starving on a cellular level. In essence, when we eat dead food, we lower our life force and vibrational frequency, which over time can lead to illness, fatigue, and emotional imbalance.

Our connection to food is sacred. It is not merely fuel but information for our cells—an energetic blueprint that communicates directly with our DNA. Eating nutrient-dense, colorful foods in their most natural form reminds the body of its inherent wisdom and ability to heal.

By returning to nature's rhythm and eating food as close to its original form as possible, we begin to restore harmony within ourselves. This isn't about perfection or deprivation—it's about awareness. Each conscious food choice becomes an act of self-love, fueling not just our body but also our mind and spirit.

So, how toxic are we? There is simply no way to sugar-coat this message. We are being poisoned by the air we breathe, the foods we eat, the water we drink, radiation, electromagnetic frequencies (EMFs), and the many household items we use daily. The good news is we can significantly minimize our exposure to toxins once we know what they are. Healthier choices will be provided for each hazard listed. Even minor tweaks and changes made over time will help. By working on protecting our health we can mitigate the dangers. Our bodies are resilient; however, with increased exposure from multiple sources, our immune systems simply cannot keep up with the work. Everything we can do to help our health today will pay off in the long run. This is a huge task. Don't get discouraged. Taking baby steps is better than not taking any. Strive for progress, not perfection.

Let's compare our health with this analogy: We purchase a fixer-upper home with amazing potential. We first clear out all the dirt, junk, and clutter, fix what's broken, give it a good scrubbing, add a fresh coat of paint, and clear out any stale, old, negative energies by burning sage, palo santo, or other energy clearing methods. We then remodel the home and fill it with beautiful, vibrant furnishings, fixtures, and decor. And lastly, to maintain the home's health and vitality, we regularly vacuum and mop the floors, take out the trash, clean the sinks and toilets, wash the windows, etc. As with our bodies, we wouldn't put quality, new furniture in a filthy, decrepit home without first cleaning it out. The following section will cover how to first remove the junk, clutter, and toxins from our body and environment, so we don't pollute it further. And then, we can decorate it and make it sparkle by eating the right foods.

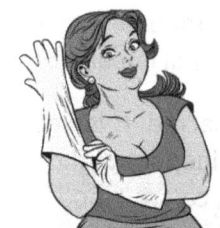

The best defense is a good offense. Let the Cleanup Begin!

Chapter 2
Removing Toxins in Our Diet

"Don't Dig Your Grave with Your Own Knife and Fork" -Old English Proverb

To properly nourish our physical, mental, and emotional bodies, we will want to eliminate all food, drink, sounds, visual stimuli, thoughts, and words that are connected to low vibrational, fear-based energy, starting with removing foods that vibrate in low frequencies. These foods are described as toxic, dead foods. They are chemically processed and devoid of all life energy that allows us to thrive in healthy bodies. Because our bodies are electric, unnatural substances created by man are not part of the biological blueprint from which we were created. Therefore, these foods cannot be recognized by the body as a food source.

Whether you're struggling with health issues or simply trying to make small changes in your diet, there are numerous practices available to help you become the best version of yourself. The first step is to limit or remove the following toxic, dead foods from your diet so you can radiate life energy and thrive in higher vibrational frequencies.

Irradiated Foods. In a modern world on the go, the convenience of quickly popping food in the microwave oven to be cooked in minutes certainly has its advantages—or does it? Foods that have been subjected to microwave radiation may be dangerous to our health. Microwave ovens nuke food with high-frequency microwaves that force water molecules to heat up by violently vibrating them. This causes a fracturing of the molecules and reorganizes the chemical composition of the food, killing its life force. Studies have shown that cooking food with microwaves may produce cancer-causing agents, destroy its nutritional value, and reduce the food's vital energy field content by up to 90%. Research reveals that the effects of eating irradiated food include the following: long-term permanent brain damage, hormone imbalances, stomach and intestinal tumors, increase in cancer cells in human blood, immune system deficiencies, loss of memory, concentration, emotional instability, and a decrease in learning and intelligence. The cumulative effects of microwaves are gradual. Therefore, when the onset of illness occurs it is very hard to make the connection to the original cause. For these reasons, eating foods and drinks that have been heated or prepared in a microwave oven is not advised.

Air fry ovens, convection toaster ovens, and infrared ovens cook faster than conventional methods and still retain the nutritional benefits of the food being prepared. Convection uses air, while infrared is a safe form of radiation that occurs when electricity is applied to a quartz crystal, creating infrared waves. Ninja is a popular manufacturer of these appliances, as is the Breville Smart Oven.

Refined Sugar. The one thing that every doctor, nutritionist, dentist, and health care professional can agree upon is that consuming refined sugar is a health hazard. Refined sugar comes from sugarcane and sugar beets, which are processed to extract the sweet flavor of sugar. Refined sugar contains no nutrition for the body. During its manufacture, sugar becomes unnatural, devitalized, demineralized, and robbed of any life-giving qualities it once possessed. Sugar robs mineral and energy reserves from the body while giving nothing in return. Our favorite sweets and delicious treats that provide us with comfort, happiness, and celebration can be addicting and, according to studies, a primary cause of over 140 diseases that are directly related to its consumption, including diabetes, heart disease, cancer, fatty liver disease, digestive issues, dementia, depression, mood swings, anxiety, acne, wrinkled skin, pain and inflammation, fatigue, obesity, infertility, impotence, poor sleep, and hormonal disruptions, to name a few.

Refined sugar is not only in the sweet treats. It is in nearly every processed food we eat and drink. The average American unknowingly consumes about 152 pounds of sugar a year! That's roughly 22 teaspoons every day for every person in America. The average child consumes about 34 teaspoons daily, making nearly one in four teenagers prediabetic or diabetic. While brown sugar, turbinado sugar, and organic cane sugar may be slightly better options than processed white sugar, sugar is still sugar and promotes the same health problems.

Refrain from purchasing packaged snacks, cookies, cakes, donuts, etc., from the supermarkets. Limit your intake of sweet treats to special occasions. For those with a severe sweet tooth, try snacking on one ounce (square) of organic, fair-trade chocolate with 70% or higher cacao content. The goal is not to deprive ourselves but to change our habits to more favorable choices that provide the body with nutrition.

By baking our own desserts and sweet treats, we can control the type and amount of sugar in the ingredients. Some healthy sugar substitutes, such as coconut sugar and monk fruit sweetener, have the same 1:1 ratio as the original recipe that calls for sugar.

Substituting sugar with natural alternatives not only sweetens your foods and beverages but may also add some health benefits. Experiment with several options for different needs from the following list: monk fruit sweetener, allulose, coconut sugar, organic raw honey, authentic maple syrup, or stevia. Stevia is a nice sugar substitute for coffee and tea, although it does have a bitter aftertaste and is often less favorable for that reason.

Artificial Sugars/Chemical Sweeteners. Aspartame is a chemical used as a sugar substitute in diet sodas as well as over 5,000 food products, sugar-free chewing gums, and many beverages. It is marketed under different names such as *Sweet'N Low, Equal, Splenda,* etc. Saccharin is the chemical that makes Sweet'N Low. Sucralose is the chemical substance that makes Splenda. These types of sweeteners can be found in products that market diet foods as low-carb and sugar-free. It is also used in diabetic-approved foods as they do not cause blood-sugar spikes like refined sugar and other natural sweeteners.

All these products are synthetic compounds that can be toxic to every system of the body. It has been documented that over 90 different health-related side effects are associated with their consumption such as brain tumors, birth defects, anxiety and panic attacks, seizures, headaches and migraines, dizziness / vertigo, muscle spasms, weight gain, numbness, rashes, depression, PMS, hearing loss, breathing difficulties, slurred speech, tachycardia, tinnitus, loss of taste, hair thinning, asthma, memory loss, joint pain, confusion, tremors, restless legs, hyperactivity, peptic ulcers, fatigue, irritability, hypoglycemia, and more.

High fructose corn syrup (HFCS): HFCS is another sweetener that must be mentioned in this category. This industrial sugar substitute is used to sweeten many processed foods and beverages. It is made from corn starch and is relatively inexpensive to manufacture. HFCS has been associated with increased concentrations of uric acid in the blood, which may be linked to a higher risk of gout, high blood pressure, obesity, diabetes, kidney disease, and cardiovascular disease.

Be sure to check the labels when purchasing processed foods that are marketed as low-fat, no-fat, diet, low-calorie, low-glycemic, etc. The healthiest alternatives I have found that are low glycemic without calories is stevia, monk fruit, and allulose.

Soft Drinks/Colas. There is nothing that makes me cringe more than being behind a person at the grocery store checkout with a case or a liter bottle of their favorite carbonated poison. Simply stated, soda (or carbonated soft drinks) contains an alarming amount of sugar or artificial sweeteners, chemicals and harmful additives that have absolutely NO nutritional value. In addition, they are the most acid forming of all beverages. These acidic chemical-laden beverages contain carbonic acid and phosphoric acid, which, over time, cause demineralization of our teeth and deplete the body of essential minerals. Phosphoric acid interferes with the body's ability to use calcium, leading to osteoporosis or bone softening. It also neutralizes the hydrochloric acid in our stomach, which can interfere with digestion. Sodas generally contain caffeine which can cause jitters, insomnia, high blood pressure, irregular heartbeat, and elevated cholesterol levels. The caramel coloring is a potential carcinogen that may lead to cancer and other health hazards. Both regular and diet sodas (including brands that market their soda as natural) are hazardous to your health and should be completely eliminated.

Better alternatives to wean off soft drinks are mineral water or flavored sparkling or seltzer waters. However, the process of carbonation causes water to become acidic, so it's best to limit your intake.

The best thing we can drink throughout the day is pure, fresh water! Consider infusing your water with lemon, fruit slices, cucumber, or fresh herbs. Try making homemade lemonade with freshly squeezed lemon juice and water, sweetened with a few drops of monk fruit for a delicious and refreshing healthy treat.

Processed Foods. You can now see the trend of all our poisonous junk foods. If real foods have been altered by manufacturing plants, large money-making corporations, or laboratories, they are likely harmful to our health. Taking a natural God-given food source and changing its chemical composition by removing nutrients and adding chemical poisons to enhance flavor and extend shelf life—all for the sake of convenience to consumers and profits for the manufacturers, is an absolute health disaster.

Basically, if a food product is manufactured in a factory and is wrapped in plastic, tin, aluminum, glass, or paper, it is processed and not in the best interest of your health. Processed food, which makes up most of the world's diet, is loaded with flavor enhancers, preservatives, and artificial colorings to make it tasty, colorful, and have a long shelf life for the manufacturers. These so-called foods are processed to the extent that every scrap of natural nutrients they once contained is gone. Fortunately for the food manufacturers, many also have financial interests in Big Pharma and the medical-industrial complex. It's all very convenient to keep profits rolling in.

Some pre-packaged foods can be exceptions from what is considered processed. For example, grocers often wrap food prepared fresh that day in their kitchen. These choices are occasionally acceptable, assuming you know and understand the ingredients used in their recipes. Read the labels carefully. Some seemingly healthy choices may contain hidden ingredients such as wheat and soy.

Just say "**no**" to foods that are not real. Processed foods are stored in the center aisles of the grocery store. By shopping around the parameters of the store, you will find the fresh and refrigerated products as well as organic fruits and vegetables. Whole, natural foods will always be the best choice.

Genetically Modified Organisms (GMOs). Again, let's pick on the industrialized controllers who, through technology and innovations, are adamant about playing God with our food, environment, and bodies to change food from their beautiful, natural form to behave differently...for our benefit, of course! Or so the story goes.

Genetically altered food is food derived from plants or animals that have had their genetic structure altered by splicing in genes from another species. In other words, their DNA has been artificially manipulated. Genetic engineering is changing the composition of foods. Many countries require genetically modified foods to be labeled. The National Bioengineered Food Disclosure Standard (NBFDS), which was published in the Federal Register in December 2018, didn't require the start of mandatory GMO labeling by manufacturers in the United States until 2022. The standard mandates using the term "bioengineered" or genetically engineered (GE foods) instead of "GMO" in disclosures. GMOs have become controversial as competing narratives have emerged about the safety of the ingredients and end products. The controversy has led to a segment of consumers who do not want such products in their diet.

Scientists are experimenting with these processes in an attempt to increase yields and improve plant resistance to toxins and pests, not knowing what the long-term effects will be on our health. On paper, altered foods may appear to offer innovative solutions for farmers and consumers. But let's look a little closer. Food that has been natural since the beginning of time has now had its genetic structure changed by humans. If the food's genetic structure has changed, so has its electrical nature. The human body thrives only on natural food. It can only be nourished or recharged by electrically compatible patterns. The cells of our bodies cannot utilize unnatural, processed, altered, or distorted electrical patterns without succumbing to disease.

The most common genetically engineered food crops and end products are corn, soy, canola oil / rapeseed, Hawaiian papaya, yellow squash, zucchini, alfalfa, sugar beets, and sugar. As a byproduct, poultry, beef, eggs, and dairy from chickens and cows raised in large-scale operations or concentrated animal feeding operations (CAFOs) are fed corn and soy as well as well as injected with hormones to help them grow faster. In addition, animals raised under inhumane and unfavorable conditions release stress hormones, all of which end up in the final product. We eat what they eat. The bottom line is we can only control our own space and our own health choices. When purchasing any of these foods, choose non-GMO. it is imperative to buy these items from certified organic farms. Also, when buying and consuming chicken and beef, buy from organic, grass-fed farms. Eggs should be organic and cage-free.

> **A profound message from the Tao Te Ching – *Lao Tzu***
> Do you think you can take over the universe and improve it?
> I do not believe it can be done. The universe is sacred.
> You cannot improve it. If you try to change it, you will ruin it.
> If you try to hold it, you will lose it.

Non-Organic Foods. Non-organic foods are foods and drinks not produced by methods complying with the standards of organic farming. Standards vary worldwide, but organic farming feature practices that cycle resources, promote ecological balance, and conserve biodiversity. The average consumer believes that the primary issue of nonorganic foods correlate to pesticide residue, but there is so much more to it. The health issues of eating foods that are not organic are as follows:

Nonorganic foods are sure to contain certain pesticides and fertilizers due to the farming methods used to produce these products. Chemical pesticides and herbicides have been linked to birth defects, obesity, diabetes, ADHD, cancer, and other health problems. The Environmental Working Group (EWG) published the "Dirty Dozen" or "Dirty 12," identifying foods that are more susceptible to retaining pesticides even after washing. These are: strawberries, spinach, kale (including collard and mustard greens), apples, grapes, cherries, peaches, pears, bell peppers, celery, and tomatoes. Although not on their list, non-organic potatoes should be added as well.

Nonorganic foods are processed using irradiation, industrial solvents, or synthetic food additives. Irradiated food is exposed to intense ionizing radiation. This is done in a processing room for a specified duration. Food irradiation uses radiant energy (electrons, gamma rays, or x-rays) to break chemical bonds and reduce microorganisms. The concern is that radiation is known to cause cancer. Nonorganic farmers also produce genetically modified foods and beverages (as previously discussed). Lastly, Nonorganic foods contain artificial preservatives, colors, and flavors (as previously discussed).

Now that we have summed up why we must avoid all forms of nonorganic foods, we should probably discuss what constitutes "organic" as well as the different forms. The marketing of food and labels can be tricky with their enticing claims. In the United States, there are three levels of organic certification to the USDA's National Organic Program (NOP). A label of "100% Organic" means that all the listed ingredients (excluding water and salt) are entirely, 100% organic. An "Organic" label is given to any product that has a minimum of 95% organic content by weight. These products may contain a small number of natural preservatives or processing aids (from a list of approved ingredients) that exclude them from the 100% Organic label. A "Made with Organic" label applies to products with a minimum of 70% organic content by weight. Use your common sense when purchasing processed foods. Just because a label claims to be organic doesn't mean the product is healthy, such as "organic Doritos." Read labels carefully. They can be misleading.

Regarding agricultural products, in the U.S.A., "Certified Organic" refers to products grown and processed in accordance with the U.S. Department of Agriculture's (USDA) organic standards, followed by certification by state and private agencies accredited by the USDA. Acquiring a "Certified Organic" label is expensive and challenging to acquire due to the extensive paperwork and scrutiny of government regulations, which could exclude small organic farmers from this category. Get to know your local farmers and do your research. Your local farmers may supply some of the healthiest foods around.

Choosing organic foods and produce will ensure that more nutrients stay on your plate and that dangerous, toxic-laden chemicals and neurotoxins stay off your plate. When unsure, pay attention to the produce codes on the stickers. If it is organic, it will have a five-digit code starting with "9." A nonorganic code will only have four numbers.

Fried Foods / Junk Foods / Fast Foods. These categories encompass a wide range of foods from convenience foods, comfort foods, and America's favorites such as McDonald's French fries, fried chicken, fish and chips, Popeyes chicken sandwiches and packaged treats such as potato chips. There is quite a bit of overlap in this group which is why they are being lumped together. The purpose is not to completely discourage eating some of your favorites, but to be aware of what you're eating. It's okay to have these foods occasionally, but only in small amounts, for the following reasons:

Fried Food Risks: Fried foods are high in fat, calories, and often salt. Studies have linked fried foods to numerous serious health problems. Fried foods served in fast-food restaurants are usually cooked in hydrogenated oils, which are high in trans fats. Many restaurants use these oils because they give food a satisfying taste and crunch. Trans fats raise harmful LDL cholesterol levels and lower good (HDL), which may increase heart disease risk. Acrylamide, a cancer-causing chemical, forms in foods cooked at high temperatures when the amino acid asparagine reacts with sugars during the cooking process. This chemical can form in many fried foods, but it's especially common in potatoes, which are high in sugars like fructose and glucose. Common foods such as fried potatoes and French fries are favorites for so many people. It's no wonder that heart disease and cancer are the top two causes of death. A discussion on oils will be presented later in this section.

Junk Food Risks: Junk food got its name for a reason—it does not provide quality nutrition. In fact, it robs the body of nutrition and contributes to degenerative disease and related conditions. Eating a regular junk food diet leads to vitamin, mineral, amino acid, and enzyme deficiencies. Junk foods are "dead" because they lack live enzymes. Most of these so-called foods have been refined, processed, and overheated. To top it off, chemicals have been added as taste enhancers and preservatives. Junk food is toxic and stressful to the body and should be avoided at all costs.

Fast Food Risks: Fast food provides mass-produced, pre-prepared, chemically seasoned and processed, non-organic ingredients posing as a meal. It is an affordable and convenient way to fill yourself up when on the run. We shouldn't feel guilty for an occasional indulgence, however, regularly eating fast food can seriously damage our health. It supplies the body with very little nutrition and is high in fat, calories, and sodium, which can lead to various health issues. The most common health concerns are weight gain, obesity, diabetes, depression, and cardiovascular conditions.

By significantly reducing or avoiding these types of foods over time, the cravings will disappear, and the thought of indulging your favorites will often seem undesirable. Your tastes will change after healthy foods become a way of life. In addition, extra weight will fall off, brain fog will lift, digestion will improve, and skin will glow.

The Five White Poisons. The following foods—refined white rice, refined salt, pasteurized cow's milk, refined sugar, and white flour—are coined as the five white poisons because they contain no nutritional value and produce acid in the body. They draw on the body's nutrient resources while being digested. These foods should be limited or removed from our diets because they are health-depleting.

- **White Rice:** White rice is a staple in nearly every culture. But what we don't realize is that white rice processing involves a refining process that removes the outer layer and germ, leaving only the endosperm, which consists primarily of starch. This can significantly increase glucose levels in our bloodstream, leading to diabetes and weight gain.

Organic quinoa, brown rice, and wild rice are excellent and delicious replacements for refined white rice. Broccoli and cauliflower rice are also fun and nutritious, low-carbohydrate substitutes if calorie-cutting is a goal.

- **Table Salt:** Sodium is an essential electrolyte; however, not all sodium is created equally. Table salt—sodium chloride (NaCl)—is found at most restaurants and consumed in many homes. It has been refined, processed, and depleted of its minerals. It is toxic and addictive and contains no nutritional value. Because it cannot be metabolized and assimilated, it accumulates in the body and becomes highly acidic. Its consumption is linked to high blood pressure and hardening of the arteries. It places great stress on the kidneys and dehydrates the body as it tries to filter out excess sodium through the urine. Health hazards linked to refined salt include osteoporosis and heart disease.

Unhealthy salt can be replaced with a reputable, unrefined and unprocessed sea salt that contain loads of trace minerals. Quality sea salt will have no additives and no change in taste (except maybe for the better). They can be purchased at most stores and online. Top favorites are Redmond Real Sea Salt, Celtic Sea Salt, Himalayan Sea Salt, and Hawaiian Black Lava Sea Salt.

- **Pasteurized Cow's Milk:** Because commercial dairy products are so depleting to our health, they've earned their own category (discussed below).

- **Refined Sugar:** Sugar also earned its own category (as explained above).

- **White Flour:** A wheat seed's two most nutritious and fiber-rich parts are the outside bran layer and the germ (embryo). Highly processed white flour is missing both of these healthy components due to processing. When refined white flour is made, the bran and the germ are removed, leaving only the starchy endosperm. This makes it more shelf-stable but results in a significant nutrient loss. To meet government guidelines and regulations, the product is then fortified with synthetic vitamins and minerals that are not easily recognized by our bodies as food and therefore cannot be readily absorbed. This inferior food robs us of our nutrients to break it down. White flour can affect our health in the following ways: blood sugar spikes, diabetes, weight gain, belly fat, obesity, high LDL cholesterol, heart disease, inflammation, digestion issues, and can aid in the growth of cancer cells. White flour also contains gluten, which will be discussed subsequently. Commercial white flour is found in tortillas, bread, pasta, cereals, baked goods such as muffins, cookies, cakes, pie crusts, crackers, and pizza crusts.

Nutritious and delicious alternatives to white flour are gluten-free whole grains and nut flours such as coconut, almond, pecan, cashew, walnut, as well as seed flours such as sesame, sunflower, and pumpkin. Other excellent choices for baking include teff, sorghum, amaranth, and gluten-free oats. If you don't have a gluten sensitivity and can't live without wheat, look for organic sprouted wheat products. Raw mesquite powder is a healthy addition to recipes as a gluten-free flour substitute and offers a sweet, smoky taste with hints of caramel and maple.

Dairy. The consumption of commercial dairy products is harmful to the health of the body for several reasons. Unless milk is purchased directly from a dairy farm, it has most likely gone through a pasteurization process. The Centers for Disease Control and Prevention (CDC) states that raw milk can carry dangerous bacteria such as Salmonella, E. coli, Listeria, and Campylobacter. Therefore, the U.S. Food and Drug Administration (FDA) bans anyone from selling or distributing unpasteurized milk for human consumption via interstate commerce. Raw milk cheese (cheese made with unpasteurized milk) is also prohibited from being sold throughout the United States unless it has been aged for at least 60 days. The aging process allows the acids and salts in the cheese to naturally inhibit the growth of harmful bacteria.

Pasteurized milk contains no enzymes, is acid-forming, mucus-clogging, and challenging to digest. And although raw milk and cheese have its nutritional values intact, they are high in allergens, which can cause havoc for people with lactose or casein sensitivities. The dairy industry is a huge business. We have been led to believe through the media and governmental guidelines that we need milk for its calcium content to build strong bones. Numerous studies show that this is not only a myth but a downright lie. The high temperature of pasteurization kills enzymes in milk and denatures its minerals. The body cannot utilize unnatural minerals. The denatured calcium that the body is unable to eliminate is deposited on the outside of the bones and in between joints, where it causes bone spurs and arthritis. If it is in the tissues, it causes fibromyalgia. During the process of metabolizing and eliminating pasteurized dairy products, calcium is actually drawn out of the body. Milk was created for calves. We are the only species that continues to drink milk after we have been weaned. Even adult cows don't drink it.

The FDA, as well as the various forms of propaganda, state that milk is a healthy food item and that pasteurization does not reduce the health benefits of milk, nor does it cause allergic reactions or lactose intolerance. I have worked with enough clients and followed enough science to respectfully disagree. Many of my clients, both young and old, cannot tolerate dairy due to allergens that can cause the body to develop mucus, gas, intestinal cramps, diarrhea, constipation, skin conditions, congestion, bronchitis, ear infections, rashes, tooth decay, arthritis, asthma, and acid reflux. It is a common practice to put autistic children, as well as those with ADD, on casein and gluten-free diets as a form of treatment. Cow's milk and dairy products have also been found to be the most common culprits for infants experiencing colic or colic-like symptoms. The two main allergens in milk products are lactose and casein. Lactose intolerance is caused by a lack of the enzyme lactase needed to break down and digest the sugar in the milk. Those who are lactose intolerant often take lactase enzymes to help with the digestion of dairy. Casein (Sodium caseinate) is the cow's main protein (80%). Whey makes up the other 20%. The main difference between casein and whey is that casein is a slow-digesting protein, which can take up to eight hours for the body to digest. Without the necessary enzymes, such as chymosin, pepsin, trypsin, and leucine aminopeptidase, to break it down, casein coagulates in the stomach, making it difficult for the digestive system to break it down due to its glue-like effect. In fact, casein is an ingredient in some types of glue. Furthermore, when casein breaks down in the stomach, it produces casomorphins, which can have an opioid effect that can be addicting.

Another major issue with conventional, non-organic dairy is the fact that it is loaded with hormones and drugs to keep cows alive and functioning in order to produce high volumes. Dairy cows are treated with antibiotics, penicillin, and hormones such as recombinant bovine growth hormone (rBGH). This is what they are referring to when you see an *rBGH-free* claim on packaging labels. Basically, what the cow consumes, so do we.

In addition to the annoying symptoms dairy can have on our bodies, a famous study called *The China Study* by Dr. T. Colin Campbell, established that casein promotes cancer in all stages of its development. Further, he found that plant-based protein did not support cancer development. For these reasons, commercial dairy products must be reduced or removed from our diets.

The good news is that between nuts and seeds, there are so many delicious and healthy alternatives to commercial dairy products. Ounce for ounce, nut and seed milks have lower calories than cow's milk, and they contain more calcium and vitamin D, which are easily broken down and utilized by the body. Many nut and seed milks even contain fiber, a nutrient you won't find in cow's milk. Delicious examples of nut milks are almond, coconut (which is technically a fruit), cashew, macadamia, walnut, and hazelnut. If you are allergic to nuts, a better milk alternative would be seed-based or plant-based milks such as oat milk. Some examples of seed milks are hemp, sesame, pumpkin, sunflower, flax, and chia seeds. For an occasional treat, many dairy-free ice cream varieties are available, but remember, dairy-free ice cream also contains sugar, so eat it in moderation. Many dairy-free milks also come in powder form which makes for a good creamer for coffee or tea. MCT oil powder is a good one. Unless you are making milk from scratch, always purchase the unsweetened option.

Gourmet cheese lovers, you will have a much harder time transitioning away from dairy. However, there are some substitutes made from nuts that are delicious. Cheeses made from goat's milk are much easier for the body to digest and may be a good option. There are more than 30 types of cheeses available that are prepared with goat's milk. The difference between each type of cheese is the primary fermentation process, followed by the taste and texture of the cheese. Some of the most popular varieties are blue cheese, chèvre, Fromage Blanc, feta cheese, and robiola. It is important to look at the labels closely when purchasing items. For example, feta cheese, contrary to popular belief, are often made from cow's milk, or a combination of cow's and goat's milk. Whenever you need a cheesy sprinkle, nutritional yeast is a tasty and healthy alternative to parmesan cheese.

As a side note, I have had clients who have dairy intolerances claim that they have had no problems digesting fresh, farm-direct cow's milk. If you find it impossible to give up cheese, and do not have a health or dairy allergy, consider trying organic raw cheeses in moderation.

Wheat & Gluten. Gluten intolerance is a factor in individuals with celiac disease (an autoimmune disease in which gluten triggers the production of antibodies that attack and damage the lining of the small intestine). However, many people have a gluten sensitivity and may not even be aware of it. Common symptoms can include diarrhea, constipation, skin conditions, depression, anxiety, autoimmune disorders, joint or muscle pain, arthritis, bloating, stomach pain, headaches, and brain fog. Then there are the rest who have zero issues with wheat and gluten. Let's take a closer look at what exactly gluten is and what foods contain this substance.

Gluten is a protein complex comprised of gliadin which contains 53% of the protein complex of gluten. Glutenin is the remaining 47% of the protein complex of gluten. It is found in several grains including wheat and related grains such as semolina, bulgur wheat, durum wheat, einkorn wheat, spelt, barley, malt, rye, Kamut (Khorasan wheat), and triticale.

One may wonder why there is so much talk about gluten today as opposed to when we were kids. Basically, the wheat cultivated and grown today bears little resemblance to wheat from forty years ago. Commercial wheat has been re-engineered through crossbreeding techniques to create high-yielding crops that contain up to five times the natural gluten content. Furthermore, gluten is difficult to digest due to its glue-like nature and high lectin content (carbohydrate-binding protein).

Lectins have been condemned because they can bind to the sugars in the cell walls of the gut or the blood, impairing the lining of the GI tract, causing the intestines to become inflamed. Consequently, the tight junctions of the intestinal wall widen, allowing various undigested food particles, toxins, and bacteria to pass into the bloodstream, causing an immune response, leading to inflammation, intestinal damage, altered gut flora, malabsorption, decreased cellular repair, cellular death, and eventually disease. This disorder is referred to as leaky gut.

Changing over to a gluten-free diet is beneficial for our health, although it can be tricky because it is not only found in food products naturally made from grains; it is also used as an additive to many products to improve texture that we wouldn't expect. Some obvious and not so apparent items to avoid (unless labeled "Gluten-Free") are pasta, pizza crust, imitation meats, sauces, salad dressings, beer, ketchup, canned soups, soy sauce, gravy, crackers, cereals, ice cream, and soup bouillon cubes and broths, corn tortillas, and commercial dairy products that have grain-fed diets, to name a few. Extra gluten is also generally added to commercially produced bread as it makes the dough rise more easily and improves the texture. Sourdough bread, due to its lengthy fermentation process, is often better tolerated by individuals with gluten sensitivities than other types of bread. The fermentation breaks down gluten, making it easier to digest, according to some researchers and bakers. However, it is crucial to note that sourdough bread is not gluten-free and still contains gluten. Gluten can also be found in pet food and in various cosmetic, hair, and skin products.

Eliminating gluten from our diet can feel like a daunting task at first. Whether the goal is to feel better, eat cleaner, relieve digestive symptoms, or manage a gluten-induced illness, once a bit of homework is done, eating gluten-free still provides delicious alternatives including gluten-free pasta, breads, pizza crust, and liquid aminos (a soy sauce alternative). Even certain vodkas (made from potato) are gluten-free. Wine is naturally gluten-free. Many restaurants offer gluten-free versions on their menus. When shopping, look at labels closely for the Gluten-Free certification. To find a list of brands and items that are gluten-free, visit the Gluten Intolerance Group at www.gfco.org.

Soy & Processed Soy Products. Soy and soy products have been marketed as a healthy alternative to meat and dairy, although it may not be the wonder food it is made out to be. In fact, due to ongoing research, many believe that commercial soy products may have more unhealthy attributes than good ones. Soy is a unique food widely studied for its estrogenic and anti-estrogenic effects on the body. Studies may seem to present conflicting conclusions about soy, but this is mainly due to the wide variation in how soy is studied and by whom the studies are funded.

For a little background, soybeans were initially used in the U.S. as a commercial crop during the early 1900s. It wasn't until fat and oil imports were blocked during World War II that we actually started to eat the beans. And once the FDA approved a health claim in 1999 that consuming 25 grams of soy protein could reduce the risk of heart disease, soybean isolates were born. Commercial production and consumption of this inexpensive protein source were used in the production of energy bars, soy burgers, soy bacon, cheese, chicken-less nuggets, corn dogs, hot dogs, ice cream, and more. In addition, many packaged foods are made with soy oil and flour. These include baked goods, canned broths and soups, canned meats, cereals, crackers, sauces, gravy, soy milk, and infant formulas.

There is substantial interest in the possible anticancer effects of soy foods. In part, this is because of the historically low incidence rates of breast and prostate cancer in Asia. Isoflavones have received much attention. Awareness of this research has led to increasing consumer use of soy foods, isoflavone-fortified foods, and isoflavone supplements. Traditional Asian cultures provide a healthful model and one that is much different than ours. They only consume fermented soy products or tofu in small amounts as condiments but not as a main source of protein.

Soy in the United States is a huge business. It is the second largest crop in cash sales after corn, making America the world's leading soybean producer and exporter according to the American Soybean Association. Ninety-four percent of soybeans are GMO crops. As mentioned earlier, it changes the chemistry, which makes it hard for the body to digest. Plus, it is heavily sprayed with herbicides and contains high amounts of lectin, making soy one of the top allergenic foods in America. Soy has become the basis for many of the additives found in processed foods, such as artificial flavoring and hydrolyzed vegetable protein to soy lecithin, and soybean oil, among countless others.

The questionable soy contents are phytoestrogens, goitrogens, phytates, and trypsin inhibitors regarding their potential consequences on the body. With every study revealing the possible negative health effects, there will be a study contradicting those studies and promoting the positive attributes of soy.

Phytoestrogens are plant-based estrogens that mimic estrogen in our bodies. In recent years, you may have read about studies indicating that phytoestrogens are good for you. But guess who funded those studies? That's right, the soy industry! However, independent research has clearly shown that consuming phytoestrogens may contribute to breast cancer, endometriosis, uterine fibroids, infertility, and estrogen dominance (where estrogen outweighs the level of progesterone in the body). Further studies have shown that an infant taking the recommended amount of soy formula is consuming a hormone load equivalent of nearly five birth control pills per day! This alone is a primary reason to avoid using soy formulas. They have also been documented to cause extreme emotional behavior, asthma, immune system disorders, pituitary insufficiency, thyroid disorders, and irregular bowel movements. It has often been questioned if there is a correlation between soy formula consumption and why girls fed soy-based formulas are reaching puberty much younger than in the past.

Goitrogens work by preventing your thyroid from getting the necessary amount of iodine, which is a problem for those who have trouble with their metabolism, weight gain, unstable moods, fatigue, inability to concentrate, and those who are often cold.

Phytates are enzyme inhibitors that bind to important minerals like iron, calcium, magnesium, and zinc and limit their absorption in the digestive tract. In addition, trypsin inhibitors block the digestive enzyme needed to properly digest protein.

Soy derivatives are no better than the soy protein that goes into them. For example, soy milk is a concoction of soy protein, sugar, and vegetable oil, as well as MSG and flavorings to give it the flavor of the real foods it mimics.

In conclusion, when choosing soy foods, pay attention to quality and quantity. Soybeans are naturally hard to digest. Fermentation makes them more digestible. Fermentation also deactivates soy's natural phytic acid and enzyme inhibitors, which can affect mineral and protein absorption. Tempeh, miso, tamari and shoyu are fermented. Tofu is not fermented, but tofu doesn't affect mineral or protein absorption due to the way it's made. Processed products containing soy protein isolates, soy protein concentrate, textured vegetable protein or hydrolyzed vegetable protein, are best avoided. If you are unsure of the product, check the ingredients on the label.

Fermented soy products can be nutritious and enjoyed in small amounts. Due to the long fermentation process, the levels of phytates and other nutrient inhibitors are reduced. Fermented soy products include tempeh (made from partially cooked, fermented soybeans and formed into a cake or patty), miso (a fermented soybean paste with a salty taste and buttery texture and is commonly used in miso soup), and natto (a sticky texture, strong cheese-like smell and a strong nutty savory, somewhat salty flavor). Fermented foods, such as miso soup, in moderation, are a good source of gut-healthy probiotics which can promote healthy digestion.

Soy sauce is made from fermented soybeans. However, be aware that some brands of soy sauce are made artificially using a chemical process instead of being brewed from natural bacterial and fungal cultures. The same inferior brands may also contain MSG. Because soy sauce contains gluten, there are better alternatives that taste practically identical. Tamari is a gluten-free version of soy sauce and is often served in restaurants, if requested. Bragg's Liquid Aminos is a nice soy sauce alternative as it is a gluten-free, certified non-GMO product made from unfermented soybeans. Coconut aminos are a soy-free, gluten-free liquid condiment like soy sauce but made from the fermented sap of a coconut palm tree and sea salt. Coconut aminos can be used instead of soy sauce, Bragg's Liquid Aminos, or Tamari. However, it has a noticeable sweeter taste than the others.

Finally, edamame (green immature soybeans) has nutritional value, is unprocessed, and contains fewer of the toxins previously mentioned. However, remember that unless the beans are organic, they are a GMO product. Organic edamame can be enjoyed in moderation for those without soy allergies.

Certain Types of Fish. Seafood is a healthy choice for lean, high-quality, easily digested protein. A 3.5-ounce serving of seafood provides almost half of an adult's daily protein needs for only 100 to 200 calories. Seafood is low in saturated fat and sodium and is a rich source of many essential vitamins and minerals as well as omega-3 fatty acids, which have many beneficial health benefits.

Most of the seafood purchased in the United States comes from marine waters and aquaculture—better known as farm-raised-fish (the breeding and cultivation of fish in controlled aquatic environments such as ponds, rivers, lakes, and ocean and man-made "closed" systems on land for commercial purposes).

Marine aquaculture produces numerous species, including oysters, clams, mussels, shrimp, seaweed, and fish such as salmon, black sea bass, sablefish, and yellowtail. There are many ways to farm marine shellfish, including "seeding" small shellfish on the seafloor or growing them in bottom or floating cages. Marine fish farming is typically done in net pens in the water or tanks on land. U.S. freshwater aquaculture produces species such as catfish and trout. Freshwater aquaculture primarily takes place in ponds or other manmade systems. In theory, farmed fish could be an option to provide much-needed nutrition and protein to the world. The growing problem of pollution in the ocean and over-fishing particular species could potentially be remedied with farms. However, this method of breeding and raising fish has been documented as an unhealthy option due to its lower nutrient content and overall toxicity compared to wild-caught fish.

The first thing to know about consuming healthy fish is to understand where your fish is coming from, along with the potential heavy metal content. For example, we have all heard of the health benefits of salmon. However, if you are ordering it in a restaurant or purchasing it from a grocer, chances are it is farm-raised unless it specifically states on the menu or on the packaging that it is fresh wild-caught. If it is unclear, ask. So, why is this important and what are the effects on our health?

For starters, farm-raised fish are given antibiotics to stave off disease that result from crowded conditions. As a result, we are eating large quantities of antibiotic-filled fish. Fish farmers also treat their fish with pesticides to combat sea lice. Sea lice from fish farms kill up to 95 percent of migrating juvenile wild salmon. The pesticides used to treat sea lice in fish farms circulate throughout the ocean. Pesticides that have been banned for decades have concentrated in the fat of various marine life. This fat is used in the feed that fish farms use, and studies by the Environmental Working Group have found that cancer-causing polychlorinated biphenyls (PCBs) exist in farm-raised salmon at sixteen times the rate of wild salmon. Dibutyltin is a chemical used in PVC plastics. Dibutyltin can interfere with normal immune responses and inflammation control in both animals and humans. A 2008 study found that dibutyltin may be contributing to the rise of allergies, asthma, obesity, and other metabolic and immune disorders in humans. Researchers have also found high levels of polybrominated diphenyl ether (PBDE), a chemical used as a flame retardant, in farm-raised fish. PBDEs are endocrine disruptors that are thought to contribute to cancer. Another study, conducted at the State University of New York at Albany, found that dioxin levels in farm-raised salmon are eleven times higher than those in wild salmon. Dioxins impair the endocrine, immune, nervous, and reproductive systems, and are carcinogens. And lastly, canthaxanthin is a synthetic pigment that adds a pink color to farm-raised salmon to mimic the fresh version that gets their color naturally by feeding on krill. Canthaxanthin is a compound found in sunless tanning pills. Studies have found that canthaxanthin can affect pigments in the retina of the eye, leading to a ban on its use in the U.K., but not in the United States. The diets of farmed fish are often genetically modified, filled with toxins, and meant to fatten them up rather than grow healthy fish. There are also certain questionable and seemingly inhumane practices that are sometimes employed in these operations. In addition to the toxic content of farm-raised fish, compared to wild-caught, farm-raised seafood, contains less omega-3s, vitamins, carotenoids, and minerals.

Another potential concern with consuming certain fish is their high content of heavy metals. The most common heavy metals that contaminate seafood are lead, cadmium, arsenic, and mercury. For many people, the primary concern is methylmercury, which forms from inorganic mercury that our bodies cannot metabolize. Inorganic mercury originates from industrial waste, smokestack emissions, volcanic activity, and coal-fired power plants. Exposure to methylmercury in food can cause neurological and behavioral issues such as anxiety, insomnia, mood swings, memory issues, tremors, headaches, depression, numbness, joint pain, trouble breathing, vision and speech impairment, muscle weakness, difficulty chewing or swallowing, and decreased immune and reproductive function as well as problems with your kidneys, lungs, digestive tract, or cardiovascular system. Because mercury can cross the blood-brain barrier, it has been linked to brain dysfunction, Alzheimer's, dementia, and autism. It can also cross the placental barrier, causing brain damage to fetuses and young children. Therefore, it is essential to understand the safe limits of the amount and types of seafood you consume.

Mercury levels differ between species due to factors such as the type of fish, size, location, habitat, diet, and age. Fish that are larger and older, and that eat other fish are at the top of the food chain contain more mercury. Depending on the weight of a person, certain fish can safely be consumed in small amounts a couple of times per week.

The following are rough safety guidelines for fish consumption regarding mercury content and how the body is able to break down the metals by body weight.

- The types of fish containing the highest levels of mercury include swordfish, shark, mackerel, snapper, tilefish, and orange roughy, and should never be eaten by *anyone,* regardless of body weight. If these types of fish have been consumed in large amounts or frequently, I recommend taking a chelating agent to help detoxify heavy metals from the body, especially mercury. Mercury accumulates in the body and brain, which can cause serious health issues; therefore, it is best to be proactive in this area.

- Seabass, marlin, grouper, trout, tuna, and lobster that may only be consumed by people weighing 175 pounds, limiting consumption to 3.5 ounces per week.

- Bluefish, halibut, cod, mahi-mahi, and Dungeness crab may be consumed by people weighing 150 pounds or more, limiting consumption to five to six ounces per week.

- Perch, canned tuna, blue crab, haddock, whitefish, and herring may be enjoyed by people weighing 100 pounds or more limiting consumption to five ounces per week.

- And lastly, King crab, catfish, scallops, sole, flounder, salmon, tilapia, clams, shrimp and oysters may be safely enjoyed by people weighing 50 pounds or more twice a week, limiting consumption to eight ounces per week.

As you can see, wild-caught salmon is an excellent choice if you are a fan of fish. It is very high in omega-3 fatty acids. And, because our bodies don't produce them, we must obtain them through our diet. Wild-caught salmon also has a healthy balance of omega-3 to omega-6 fatty acids. When you have too many omega-6 fatty acids in your body, inflammation occurs. In addition, cold water fish such as salmon are a good source of vitamin D, an extremely important nutrient essential for a wide variety of bodily functions. The sun is your best source of vitamin D, but since most people don't get enough sun in the winter months, wild-caught salmon is a great way to add more of it into your diet. Wild-caught salmon provides healthy protein, selenium, niacin, vitamin B12, phosphorus, magnesium, and vitamin B6.

Monosodium Glutamate (MSG). Monosodium glutamate (MSG) is the world's most widely used flavor enhancer and preservative. It's a little seasoning with a big problem. For that reason, it gets a special mention in the foods to avoid section. To this day, it is the topic of several debates both in the health and food production industries. Some debunk its alleged dangers and call it nonsense, while others say to avoid it like the plague. If you go to Amazon and enter a search for "MSG," you will see many brands with 4–5-star ratings from thousands of buyers. But first, what is it, and who should we believe?

MSG is a manufactured crystal powder that enhances flavor in cooking. It is the sodium salt of glutamic acid created when sodium and glutamate are combined through the fermentation of starch, sugar beets, sugar cane, or molasses.

It all began in 1908, when a Japanese chemist found a flavorful ingredient in seaweed. He later experimented with it and created a synthetic version in the lab. He later partnered with an iodine manufacturer and marketed it using the name Ajinomoto, now the world's largest producer of MSG and, interestingly, is also a drug manufacturer.

It is estimated that Americans unknowingly consume about half a gram of MSG every day, and many people may unknowingly suffer from its effects. It is unknown why the body metabolizes glutamate more efficiently than MSG. Some suspect the probable causes of MSG-induced symptoms may be related to the sodium-potassium imbalance or the absence of enzymes necessary to metabolize the sodium-rich anion form of glutamic acid through normal channels.

Although the U.S. Food and Drug Administration lists MSG as "generally recognized as safe" (GRAS), health experts believe that it can negatively affect our health and remains a heated and controversial subject depending on who you ask. Common side effects that have been reported as related to MSG consumption include severe headache, flushing, sweating, facial tightness, heart palpitations, chest pain, shortness of breath, nausea, muscle weakness; and numbness, tingling or burning in the mouth and around the face and limbs, weight gain, and inflammation.

Further, MSG acts as a neurotransmitter in the brain, which means it carries messages from one part of the brain to another. It's also known as an "excitotoxin," meaning it stimulates cells to initiate various brain processes. Some experts believe it overstimulates cells to the point of exhaustion and neuron death, causing brain damage and thereby, potentially triggering or worsening Alzheimer's disease, Parkinson's disease, Lou Gehrig's disease, and learning disabilities. An in-depth analysis of the dangers of food additives and their effects can be found in Dr. Russell Blaylock's book entitled *Excitotoxins: The Taste that Kills*.

If you look up monosodium glutamate in Wikipedia, it clearly states, "*It is a popular myth that MSG can cause headaches and other feelings of discomfort.*" However, scientific studies, medical doctors, and articles published by the Mayo Clinic say otherwise. Throughout the years, even though numerous studies have been performed, there still seems to be inconclusive evidence to verify these claims. Perhaps it is because many studies have been carried out by the International Glutamate Technical Committee (yes, that is an actual thing!), who have a vested interest in proving MSG is safe. At the very least, scientists acknowledge that certain people may be glutamate sensitive.

It is challenging to find any canned or packaged food items that do not contain MSG in one of its hidden forms. Pre-made salad dressings and gravies can be expected to contain MSG unless clearly labeled otherwise. Certain brands of chips and chip dips, including Doritos, commonly list more than one ingredient that contains MSG. Most pre-made soups, broths, and stocks contain MSG. Frozen meals, frozen pizza, ramen, instant noodles, and even some processed cheeses may include this flavor enhancer. Although MSG is considered a seasoning itself, manufacturers commonly add it to other products that are also used for seasoning. Many spice blends will include MSG in their mix. Soy sauce will always contain a naturally occurring form of MSG. Companies producing sandwich dressings like ketchup and mayonnaise tend to include MSG in their recipes. Some soft drinks, iced tea mix, and sports drinks contain MSG. This flavor enhancer can also be found in children's snacks. Some granola bars, fruit snacks, candy, gum, and some candy bars, will contain it. Even snacks most people consider healthy, such as yogurt and cottage cheese, may include MSG. This is a perfect example of why buying organic is essential. Organic food regulations provide some protection. MSG is banned from organic food. However, yeast and yeast extracts are permitted as additives in organic foods, therefore there may be some MSG in organic foods that use yeast, or yeast extract. In addition, glutamate occurs naturally in some foods that are grown organically and can cause a sensitivity for some people.

It appears that the FDA condones food producers hiding MSG In their products by allowing disguised names on food labels. The manufacturers of processed foods know that many people don't want to consume MSG because of the side effects yet are unwilling to remove it from their products because it enhances the flavor. The term MSG or monosodium glutamate is seldom seen listed on food labels. Product brands and manufacturers often disguise this additive to confuse buyers. Some common nicknames for MSG are hydrolyzed vegetable protein, autolyzed vegetable protein, textured vegetable protein, anything "glutamate", hydrolyzed yeast extract, autolyzed yeast extract, plant protein extract, sodium caseinate, calcium caseinate, yeast extract, flavor enhancer, textured whey protein, and textured soy protein. Because food manufacturers must declare when MSG is added, its food additive code number 621 will display in the ingredient list on the label of packaged foods.

Unfortunately, MSG is also widely marketed to and used in restaurants to enhance the flavors in their recipes. If you have ever eaten Chinese food high in MSG and suddenly developed a headache or a sudden onset of heart palpitations, you have likely experienced what has been coined as *Chinese Restaurant Syndrome,* which has been validated in several studies. Although Chinese restaurants are certainly not the only restaurants that use this food enhancer. It is a common fact that fast foods and chain restaurants such as McDonald's, Burger King, Taco Bell, Wendy's, TGIF, Chili's, Applebee's, Denny's, Kentucky Fried Chicken, among others, all use ingredients that have MSG in them. Because it is disguised under a different name, they will often deny using MSG. Interestingly, MSG is sold by its real name as a savory seasoning in stores and popular shopping sites such as Amazon without camouflaging its name. It gets substantial sales and great reviews from its users about how well it makes the flavor of any bland dish come to life. As you can see, there is a mixed bag of awareness.

In conclusion, MSG is the single most controversial food ingredient known to mankind. It is highly unlikely that one ingredient would get such a bad rap if it weren't unhealthy. Regardless of whether a sensitivity exists, it is best to err on the safe side and limit or avoid this food enhancer at all costs. Fast foods, low-quality corporate restaurants, and processed foods are not concerned about producing healthy products. They are profit-driven entities and only care about sales and creating a tasty product to increase profits for their shareholders.

The desire for health-conscious individuals to eliminate or avoid MSG in their diets should be a no-brainer. Meals can easily be prepared without this toxic flavor enhancer. With a bit of research and experimentation, preparing meals with whole foods is much healthier and will provide better overall flavor. Spices like a pinch of high-quality sea salt, garlic, ginger, and organic herbs naturally enhance the taste of meals and will also provide added health benefits. Cutting out fast, processed, and packaged foods as a general practice will eliminate a lot of time spent on research and label scrutiny.

Alcohol. Before we get into the health issues with alcohol, let's first touch on whether alcohol lowers our vibrational energy. The answer is, "it depends." If you are a light drinker and enjoy an occasional glass of wine with a friend, with dinner, or to relax after a hard day, and drink responsibly, chances are the answer is *no*. This demonstrates a healthy relationship with alcohol. Alternatively, if one abuses it, regularly overconsumes, gets drunk and boisterous, becomes aggressive, or starts fights, the answer absolutely, **yes.** These traits demonstrate low vibrational frequency and can lead to addiction, health problems, poor judgment, and fatal accidents.

While most of my health-conscious clients never touch alcohol, even casual drinkers need to understand a few things. Alcohol is a toxic chemical. While the liver does most of the hard work processing alcohol and removing it from our system, every organ in the body is affected that comes into contact with it. Alcohol is considered an anti-nutrient. It pulls vitamins and minerals, such as calcium, out of our bodies to process it, causing it to be bone-depleting. It is dehydrating, which causes a plethora of health issues, including wrinkles. It is acidic to the body, causing another set of issues, including digestive issues. Regular use of alcohol can contribute to glucose intolerance and obesity.

For these reasons alcohol should be limited. If it is not realistic or desirable to avoid it completely, then choose wisely. Wine has some antioxidant properties. Consuming wine is acceptable as long as there are no food intolerances to grapes, alcohol, sulfites, or tannins. Even though wine is fermented, it does contain sugar, although it's not as hard on our livers as hard alcohol.

The most toxic alcohols are the distilled ones, which include tequila, rum, and beer. They are the worst for causing sugar imbalances. Also, keep in mind that, although beer does not contain sugar, it is high in calories and contains gluten.

The recommended healthy range for drinkers is one drink per day for women (one ounce of hard alcohol or a six-ounce glass of wine) and two for men.

In conclusion, wine, in moderation, is the best choice when drinking alcohol, particularly red wine, if your body can tolerate tannins. If possible, it is best to choose organic or biodynamic brands with no added sulfites. Wine is naturally gluten-free. If you prefer a cocktail or martini, your best choice is vodka. Even if made with wheat, barley, or rye, distilled vodka is considered gluten-free. Try to choose an organic brand when possible.

Caffeine & Coffee. Caffeine is in the alkaloid family (a class of naturally occurring compounds that mostly contain basic nitrogen atoms that can be potentially toxic for some people) consisting of a bitter substance occurring naturally in over sixty plants including coffee beans, tea leaves, kola nuts, which are used to flavor soft drinks and colas, and cacao pods, which are used to make chocolate products. A synthetic version also exists, which is added to some medicines, foods, and drinks. For example, some pain relievers, cold medicines, and over-the-counter alertness aids contain synthetic caffeine. Caffeine is also abundant in energy drinks and energy-boosting snacks.

More than 90% of adults in the United States regularly consume caffeine, averaging about 200 mg of caffeine per day. One 8-oz cup of coffee contains approximately 120 mg of caffeine. Yerba mate and guayusa teas may contain more caffeine than a cup of coffee, measuring in at 180mg per cup. Red Bull contains up to 80mg, matcha tea contains around 70mg, black tea has 40-70mg, and green tea has 35-45mg of caffeine. Oolong tea contains between 37–55 mg. Coca-Cola Classic and most caffeinated colas are in the 34 mg range. White tea contains the least caffeine of around 15-30 mg.

Soon after caffeine is consumed, it's absorbed through the small intestine and dissolved into the bloodstream. Due to its stimulant nature, it causes the body to increase its metabolism. The central nervous system becomes stimulated, so coffee drinkers feel more awake by creating a false sense of energy. Upon ingestion, the body interprets caffeine as an alkaloid poison. To rid itself of this perceived toxin, the body draws energy and minerals from its emergency reserves. In this process, stomach temperature is raised, stomach acid increases, sometimes leading to an upset stomach or heartburn, enzyme production is decreased, digestion becomes difficult, heart rate is increased, blood vessels in the brain become narrower, lungs work harder, the nervous system is irritated, and the adrenal glands, liver and pancreas are stressed. Caffeine is a diuretic, causing the kidneys to produce more urine. It also interferes with calcium absorption in the body and increases blood pressure. Although caffeine levels peak in the blood within one hour, the body may continue to feel the effects for up to eight hours.

Like alcohol, coffee is dehydrating and acidic to the body. Although coffee contains antioxidant properties, the health risks may outweigh the benefits. In addition, unless an organic roast is consumed, the chances are you are also consuming harmful pesticides. For individuals treating or recovering from any type of illness, because both caffeine and alcohol inhibit the healing process, I recommend eliminating both substances to conserve vital digestive energy for healing instead of creating more work for the body to remove these toxins.

There are ongoing debates as to whether caffeine is addictive, however, when coffee drinkers try to go off it cold turkey, a caffeine withdrawal is likely, which can be mild to extreme. Caffeine withdrawal is a medically recognized condition that occurs when people experience significant symptoms after abruptly quitting caffeine consumption. These symptoms typically appear within a day of quitting and can last a week or more. Symptoms of caffeine withdrawal include headaches, irritability, fatigue, anxiety, difficulty concentrating, depressed mood, tremors, and low energy. It is suggested that people who would like to quit do it slowly over time and drink extra water to help lessen the symptoms.

If you genuinely enjoy the flavor of coffee and as long as there are no symptoms or allergies associated with caffeine, an occasional cup in the morning is acceptable and should be out of the bloodstream before bedtime and should not disrupt sleep cycles. However, if black coffee is not your thing, then wise choices need to be made, such as a healthy sweetener and creamer. Refer to the Sugar and Dairy sections for recommendations. In addition, fresh ground, organic coffees are always best. For those striving for optimal health but still want a hot morning beverage without the caffeine, you're in luck. There are many healthy caffeine-free substitutes from which to choose. However, decaffeinated coffee is not one of them.

Decaffeinated coffee is not recommended due to the synthetic, toxic chemicals used in the extraction process. Although in 1999, the FDA concluded that the trace amounts you get in decaf coffee are too minuscule to affect your health, I choose to pass. The decaffeination process begins with unroasted beans immersed in water for a few hours to dissolve the caffeine. The chemicals methylene chloride (used for paint removal) or ethyl acetate (utilized in nail polish remover and glue removal products) extract caffeine from the water by mixing them into the water and coffee beans. The water is then evaporated to ensure the flavor stays inside the beans. Other safer methods can be used to remove caffeine from the beans, such as the Swiss water process and liquid carbon dioxide; however, most commercial roasters use the chemical-based removal and don't specify the method of extraction process used, nor is it required on the labeling.

Plenty of caffeine-free alternatives for that morning cup of coffee are available. There will be a period of trial and error. Be patient and keep trying until you are satisfied with your discovery. Teeccino offers a large assortment of brewable herbal coffees that are made with healthy chicory, contains no acid, and naturally boosts energy. This brand offers a variety of flavored coffees and teas. Pero and Kaffree Roma are instant caffeine-free, acid-free coffee substitutes added to hot water. They are made with barley, chicory, and rye. Herbal teas such as chamomile, ginger, and peppermint are naturally caffeine-free. This is because these types of teas are not made from the Camellia sinensis plant, as most teas are. Instead, they are made from dried flowers, leaves, fruits, seeds, or generally caffeine-free roots. Rooibos tea is another herbal tea that is loaded with antioxidants and worth exploring. And finally, hot water with fresh lemon juice is a refreshing and healthy way to start the day.

Hydrogenated Oils and Trans Fats. Now it's time to pick on hydrogenated oils. While it is important to incorporate healthy fats and oils into our diet, it is just as important to remove the harmful fats and oils.

As you can guess, hydrogenated oil is chemically altered by food manufacturers to keep foods fresher longer. There are two types of hydrogenated oils: partially hydrogenated (PHOs), and fully hydrogenated. Through the hydrogenation process, hydrogen is added to vegetable oil forming trans fat, which has been discovered to cause serious health complications such as heart disease, stroke, type 2 diabetes, and inflammation.

Fortunately, the Food and Drug Administration (FDA) conceded that trans fats pose a potential threat to consumers. In 2015, the FDA declared the byproduct of trans fat is not "generally recognized as safe" and had to be phased out by 2018, stating as follows: "PHOs are the primary dietary source of artificial trans fat in processed foods. Removing PHOs from processed foods could prevent thousands of heart attacks and deaths each year. It's important to note that trans fat will not be gone entirely from foods because it occurs naturally in small amounts in meat and dairy products and is present at very low levels in other edible oils.

Since then, the FDA graciously extended its deadline to January 1, 2020, so that the manufacturers have more time to filter out their inventory, allowing these foods on the shelves to not go to waste. Who says they don't have a heart?

Today, manufacturers have replaced partially hydrogenated oils with a combination of oils, including fully hydrogenated oils. Fully hydrogenated oils contain much less of the dangerous trans fats. Although these fully hydrogenated oils can solve the legal trans fat issue for manufacturers, they are being created through a process called interesterification. This process removes the fatty acids from one triglyceride molecule and transfers them to another to modify the melting point and to create an oil more suitable for deep frying or making margarine with good taste and low saturated fat content. This process is sometimes marketed as an enzymatic alternative that functions much like other shortening products but with low or no trans fats and lower saturated fat. While interesterification offers very little trans fat in a final product that performs well, the process is viewed by consumers as a GMO swap solution that might one day prove to be no better than partially hydrogenated oils. Natural food advocates like the Weston A. Price Foundation are opposing the use of interesterification because it alters the molecular structure of the oils, thereby creating a substance that the body is not familiar with.

To summarize, hydrogenated oils are mostly found in packaged foods, which are best avoided. If eating the following foods, pay close attention to the labels on these products: breakfast cereals, vegetable shortening, microwave popcorn, fried food, pie crusts, pastries, potato chips, canned frosting, crackers, non-dairy coffee creamers, frozen pizza, and fast foods. Contrary to what we have been led to believe through marketing campaigns, margarine is not a healthy substitute for butter. Margarine is unhealthy and should be eliminated and replaced with organic butter or ghee. Read labels and opt for organic brands that make oils from coconuts, avocados, or olives.

But what about vegetable oils? They sound healthy, right? After all, the word *vegetable* is in the title. Unfortunately, vegetable oils are referred to as refined, bleached, deodorized oils (RBD for short) in which ongoing studies have published that certain vegetable oils like corn oil, canola oil, soybean oil, cottonseed, palm, and peanut oils deliver an excessive amount of omega-6 fatty linoleic acids and not enough omega-3 fatty acids which may be a leading cause of inflammation in the body and may lead to heart complications. It is relatively inexpensive for restaurants to use when frying. We all love our French fries, but let's try to consume fewer when eating out. Also, next time a recipe calls for vegetable oil, consider substituting it with a healthier option, such as applesauce, coconut oil, avocado oil, or organic grass-fed butter. When frying or cooking with high heat, use the following refined oils (as opposed to cold-pressed oils): avocado oil, olive oil, or coconut oil. Butter, lard, or beef tallow may also be used for cooking with heat. The cold-pressed versions are excellent choices when not cooking with heat and preparing cold dishes or salad dressings.

Unhealthy Proteins: Plant-based Meat Alternatives (PBMAs). Many believe that plant-based meat can be healthier for us (and the environment) than real meat. And, of course, their marketing makes it sound nutritious. Please don't buy into it! They are ultra-processed, which is generally associated with high amounts of sodium, added sugar, and saturated fat. According to a recent study published in December of 2024 in *Food Frontiers*, PBMAs are associated with increased depression, inflammation, and higher blood pressure, as well as lower levels of a substance tied to low levels of high-density lipoprotein, or "good" cholesterol.

The popular commercial brands that you can find in grocery stores and restaurants contain harmful ingredients such as soy, corn, gluten, and the additives mentioned above that will do more harm than good for your health. When it comes to food, if you can't pronounce it and it's not found in nature, you don't want to eat it. When dining out, always ask the server if their veggie burger patty is made in-house. If the answer is yes, it will likely be nutritious and contain delicious whole food ingredients such as black beans, quinoa, nuts or mushrooms. There are also many good recipes on the internet for veggie burgers that you can experiment with.

Factory-farmed Animal Products. It is highly recommended that all commercial, factory-farmed animal products be eliminated from our diets. The conditions are harsh and cruel. It is safe to say that all industrial farms whose goal is to provide an end-product with the best profits for their shareholders are using growth hormones and antibiotics to make livestock grow faster and survive the crowded, unsanitary conditions of factory farms to keep them plump and disease-free. It is believed that our bodies also absorb what they have been fed and injected with, as well as their stress hormones from these unsuitable conditions. All fast-food establishments and many chain restaurants serve these relatively inexpensive, inferior products, unless otherwise noted on their menu selections. Subsequently, the world-famous *China Study* suggests that a diet rich in animal products, including meat, is linked to a higher risk of chronic diseases, and advocates for a predominantly whole-food, vegan diet to reduce or reverse the development of illness.

In Summary, this chapter demonstrates that ever since industrialization become involved with all aspects of food manufacturing, food has moved further away from nature, thereby changing its composition. Processed food removes essential enzymes, minerals, and nutrients, leaving us with very little nutrition. With all the added preservatives and chemicals in today's food supply, it's no wonder our health continues to decline. The close relationship between the food and pharmaceutical industries often creates a cycle in which nutrient-poor diets contribute to chronic illness, while those very illnesses fuel the demand for medications and treatments. Understanding this connection empowers us to make more conscious choices about the foods we eat and take a proactive role in our own well-being. Those unaware of these facts and continue to eat the Standard American Diet (SAD) retain more polluted bodies, and imbalances occur. When the body is in chronic misalignment, it tends to become more and more obese, ill, and emotionally devoid—shut off from its divine intuition and Source energy. In other words, our diet affects the body, mind, and soul because everything is connected. On the positive side, learning about health and turning things around is never too late. In fact, naturopathic cancer clinics and destination programs such as the *Hippocrates Health Institute* and *Ann Wigmore Natural Health Institute*, along with many others, have helped people riddled with cancer completely heal simply by transitioning to a healthy, nutrient-dense diet.

Chapter 3
Read the Labels!

As a fun exercise, I thought it would be a good idea to randomly choose one food product from the industrialized/processed foods category and discuss the importance of reading labels. I have chosen one of my childhood favorites, the toasted Pop-Tart. Theoretically, it could be marketed as a healthy treat because it is filled with what used to be a healthy piece of fruit before the factory got hold of it. Yet that couldn't be further from the truth. Here is the list of ingredients. How many health offenders can you identify?

> **Ingredients**: Enriched flour (wheat flour, niacin, reduced iron, vitamin B1 [thiamin mononitrate], vitamin B2 [riboflavin], folic acid), corn syrup, high fructose corn syrup, dextrose, sugar, soybean and palm oil (with TBHQ for freshness), bleached wheat flour. Contains 2% or less of wheat starch, salt, dried strawberries, dried pears, dried apples, leavening (baking soda), citric acid, gelatin, modified wheat starch, yellow corn flour, color, xanthan gum, cornstarch, turmeric extract color, soy lecithin, red 40, yellow 6, blue 1, color added.

Here are the main offenders:

1. **Enriched flour**: Research has shown that consuming products made with enriched flour could be linked to an increased risk of health conditions such as obesity, type 2 diabetes, and heart disease due to its effect on blood sugar levels and lack of essential nutrients.

2. **High-fructose corn syrup** (HFCS), an artificial sugar made from corn syrup, can lead to serious health issues.

3. **Corn syrup**, a byproduct of HFCS, has been identified to cause obe-

sity, liver disease, digestive issues, heart disease, diabetes and kidney stones.

4. **Dextrose** is a chemically processed type of sugar derived from corn starch, rice, or wheat is known for raising blood sugar and may cause poor health if used regularly.

5. **Sugar**. Processed, no doubt. Where to start...

6. **Soybean oil**: hydrogenated oils should be avoided whenever possible due to a number of potential health risks.

7. **Palm oil**: Some research suggests palm oil may contribute to cancer because of the acrylamide (a substance possibly linked to cancer risk) created through glycerol (an alcohol) breakdown when palm oil is cooked in high temperatures.

8. **TBHQ**, which stands for "tertiary-butylhydroquinone", is an additive to preserve processed foods. One government study published that this additive increased the incidence of tumors in rats. Also, vision disturbances have been reported in humans.

9. **Bleached wheat flour**: Chemicals like chlorine gas or benzoyl peroxide are used to whiten the product removes the natural nutritional benefits. It is also high in gluten,

10. **Citric acid**: A synthetic additive to many packaged foods and some supplements as well as cleaning agents. Because it is produced from a type of mold, it can cause adverse reactions in some people.

11. **Modified wheat starch**: In processed foods, it may be combined with unhealthy additives, affecting digestive health; allergen; high in gluten.

12. **Yellow corn flour**: According to various health experts, corn flour is rich in carbohydrates and has a high glycemic index, causing a spike in blood sugar levels. Commercial corn is also a GMO product.

13. **Caramel coloring**: A carcinogen (a substance that may cause cancer).

14. **Soy lecithin**: Made from made from genetically modified soy. it is often extracted using chemical solvents such as hexane, a solvent made from crude oil.

15. **Red 40**: A carcinogen. Red Dye 40 is a synthetic color additive made from petroleum. This dye may be linked to allergies, migraines, and mental disorders in children. Other studies show it as a carcinogen. Many people can be unknowingly allergic to this dye as well. (Note: the FDA recently banned red dye No. 3 due to its potential cancer-causing effects. Yet, the manufacturers were given two years before it needs to be removed from their products.

16. **Yellow 6**: A carcinogen. The food coloring yellow dye #6 (Sunset Yellow) is an unhealthy additive that provides no nutritional value and numerous harmful side effects.

17. **Blue 1**: A carcinogen. Also known as "brilliant blue." Unlike the other food dyes, it crosses the blood-brain barrier. It may cause nerve cells to malfunction and contribute to chromosomal damage, allergic reactions and behavioral changes.

Yum…my fond memories of this delicious, toasted treat with melted butter on top, were nothing more than a chemical concoction with no nutritional value.

The industry rules governing label content are complicated. The marketing rules can be tricky because some offenders may be labeled as something other than what it is to confuse the consumer. The best rule of thumb would be to avoid packaged foods altogether. If this is not an option, purchase products with a "Certified Organic" symbol on the packaging.

Fortunately, technology is here to save the day. There are several very good phone apps that can scan food labels and barcodes and give you nutritional information, ingredient breakdowns, and health-quality ratings. The Yuka app is good for fast "should I consider this" while at the grocery store. It is especially helpful when shopping packaged groceries.

If you would like to dig further into the deception within the food industry, there is an interesting book titled "Feeding You Lies" by Vani Hari. If you would like pragmatic instruction of reading food labels, try "Nutrition (Know What You're Buying: How to Read Food Labels)" by C.D. Shelton.

Chapter 4
Limiting Toxins from Our Homes

Now that we have discussed how to clean up our diets, let's continue with the toxic chemical soup we absorb through our skin and lungs. We are exposed to nearly 85,000 types of harmful chemicals each day from plastics, air pollution, perfumes, cosmetics, household cleansers, dust mites, molds, solvents, fragrances, aerosol sprays, paints, and EMFs, just to name a few. While we can't do much about the environmental toxins we breathe, there is a lot we can do to detoxify our homes by using safer personal household products. Each product by itself is unlikely to cause hazardous health effects. The body is designed to flush out poisons under proper conditions, such as eating healthy, drinking enough water, and keeping our immune system operating optimally. However, the culmination of hundreds of potential chemicals entering our body is taxing to our health. If our detoxification pathways become overburdened, the potential for disease is increased. We don't always know how and why our bodies react to certain toxins. While studies reveal the common dangers, some people are more susceptible to certain risks than others. With every commercial product we use, we can replace it with a more natural, easy-to-find product. Whatever we can do to limit our exposure to toxic chemicals, the better off we will be.

Under the current law, the FDA has little authority in the United States to review chemicals in cosmetics, personal care, or household products. Manufacturers of these products are not required to register with the FDA, provide the FDA with ingredient statements, adopt Good Manufacturing Practices (GMPs), report adverse events to the FDA, or provide the FDA with access to safety records. So, it is up to us to do our own research and improve our buying habits. The categories below provide better alternatives to commercial brands.

Commercial Toiletries. The skin is our body's largest organ. Everything we apply to it gets absorbed into our bloodstream. Unless our personal care products are organic and biologically friendly, they may contain toxic ingredients. The Environmental Working Group estimates that about 20 percent of chemicals used in cosmetics could cause cancer. Yet these cancer-causing toxins are given a free pass because, in and of themselves, a single product may not pose a threat. However, multiple products used simultaneously may infuse the bloodstream with thousands of different chemicals with varying degrees of toxicity. In addition, cosmetics can be contaminated with heavy metals, including arsenic, cadmium, lead, mercury, and nickel. The good news is there are several products available in the cosmetics industry that contain natural and organic ingredients without the need to give up style and glamour.

We are often brand loyal to our favorite products, but they may not be loyal to us. Toxic ingredients are not just found in lower-priced items like Revlon or Maybelline but in the very expensive designer products as well. Brands such as Versace, Prada, Gucci, Dolce & Gabbana, are not excluded from selling us toxins. They just get to charge more for them.

In our morning routines alone, an average male uses up to nine personal care products such as toothpaste, mouthwash, shampoo, conditioner, soap, deodorant, lip balm, sunscreen, body lotion, and shaving products, which adds up to 85 different chemical ingredients that may contain cancer-causing carcinogens, neurotoxins (a poison which acts on the nervous system), and endocrine disruptors.

Women are at an even higher risk because more personal care products are used than men, including face soap, moisturizer, anti-aging cream, nail polish, nail polish remover, shampoo and conditioner, body washes or soaps, toothpaste, toner, powder, foundation, eyeliner, mascara, glue from fake eyelashes, perfume, and hair dye, providing a whopping average of 150 toxic chemicals. In addition, pregnant women can pass these toxins to their unborn children. Studies have detected up to 200 contaminants in the umbilical cord blood of newborns.

Explore the Environmental Working Group's website at www.EWG.org/skindeep. Commercial products such as sunscreens, skin products, hair products, nail products, makeup, fragrance, baby products, oral care, and men's products can be checked for ingredients and safety ratings. The suggestions for healthier options listed below are only a fraction of what is available on the market. Also, check on the internet and EWG's website for more suggestions.

Cosmetics. The commercial cosmetics and personal care products business is a poorly regulated multi-billion-dollar industry. There are thousands of dangerous cosmetics out there with an extensive list of chemicals and toxins known to cause diseases like cancer, severe allergies, hormone disruption, infertility, and fibroids. It's up to us to do our homework and read labels. Suggestions: Foundations, lipsticks, creams, etc.: Tarte, Rejuva Minerals, Juice Beauty, Thrive, Beauty Counter, miscellaneous organic skincare lines.

Toothpaste. Commercial toothpastes may contain ammonia, fluoride, ethanol, sodium lauryl sulfate, artificial colors and flavors, formaldehyde, mineral oil, saccharin, sugar, and PVP plastic which can be absorbed into the bloodstream, even if you don't swallow the toothpaste. Suggestions: Replace them with non-toxic brands or tooth powders. Good brands can be found at health food stores such as Essential Oxygen, Redmond Earthpaste, Tom's, Desert Essence, Shine Re-mineralizing Tooth Whitening Powder by OraWellness, David's (for remineralizing enamel), or Livfresh (for gum restoration). In addition, commercial dental floss brands are coated with plastics that can be ingested. Plastic-free versions are available on Amazon or health food stores.

Mouthwash. Ditch the Scope, Listerine, and other commercial mouthwashes. They're acidic and contain alcohol, dyes, and toxic chemicals. Suggestions: Tom's of Maine, Tooth & Gum Tonic, TheraBreath, or make your own using essential oils-one drop of tea tree, myrrh, and peppermint in a glass of water with a pinch of sea salt.

Hair Color. If using professional salons, choose Aveda or stylists offering all-natural, plant-based, ammonia-free color. For do-it-yourself (DIY) brands, Naturtint or Water Works. Henna is the most natural hair coloring product. However, there is a bit of a learning curve, and it can be more time-consuming.

Antiperspirants. Most antiperspirants contain aluminum. Aluminum has been linked with both Alzheimer's disease and breast cancer. Most manufacturers claim that there is not enough aluminum in their products to cause disease. While that may be true for a particular item, what is not considered is the amount we accumulate from other sources. Whenever we can make a change to absorb less, the better it will be for our health. There is trial and error whenever changing brands. If one doesn't work for you try another brand. Suggestions: Anything natural and aluminum-free.

Dr. Hauschka Sage Mint Deodorant, Vichy 24 Hour Dry Touch Roll-On, M3 Naturals Natural Deodorant for women and men contains magnesium and is vegan, gluten-free, cruelty-free, aluminum-free, paraben-free, and sulfate-free.

Shaving Cream. Shaving cream, as well as soaps, on drug-store shelves have a list of toxic ingredients, including phthalates, parfum, triethanolamine, parabens, and sodium lauryl sulfate. Suggestions: Dr. Bronner's shaving soap or gel, Alba Botanica, Pacific Shaving Company, Taylor of Old Bond Street, or The Art of Shaving are nice alternatives.

Nail Polish and Nail Polish Remover. Our nails are an extension of our skin, and as such, they will absorb the chemicals from polish into our bloodstream (even though the keratin on our nails may provide a bit of protection), messing with our kidneys, liver, and hormones. Although polish contains a plethora of toxic chemicals, the main ones are formaldehyde, dibutyl phthalate (DBP), and toluene. It is safe to say that there are no nail polishes that are 100% toxin-free. However, we can do much better with our choices. Suggestions: Check out ella+mila, Karma Organic, Priti NYC, Zoya, and more. Nail salons are fine using your polish instead of theirs. Many brands also sell a non-toxic nail polish remover. I have experimented with several brands and deem ella+mila's soy polish remover the winner. It's also okay to ditch the polish occasionally and to go natural. You can also purchase the "Is It Wet" nail buffer or something similar for a beautiful, clear shine.

Perfumes & Colognes. An abundance of toxic chemicals like benzaldehyde, camphor, ethyl acetate, benzyl acetate, linalool, acetone, and methylene chloride, along with 3,000 others may be lurking in your favorite perfumes, known to cause cumulative damage to internal organs if overused. Perfumes once made from natural ingredients like flowers and herbs gave way to synthetic formulations in the late 1970s and early 1980s. Today, they are approximately 95-100% synthetic and use crude or turpentine oil. It may be wise to say goodbye to your designer favorites. While it is impossible to replace your favorite fragrances with anything natural, you may find you like other scents just as much or better once you begin to experiment with healthier options. Suggestions: If you absolutely can't live without your scent, spray your favorite perfume in the air (while holding your breath) and walk into it. The mist will linger on your clothing without absorbing into your skin. Some toxic-free favorites are PHLUR Fragrance, Ellis Brooklyn, Abbott NYC, by Rosie Jane, and many more.

Sunscreens. We all love the summer and the nostalgic fragrance of coconut caressing the ocean breeze from our favorite commercial sunscreens that we grew up with. However, some of these chemical-ridden sunscreens with synthetic fragrances can cause us more harm than good. In the sunscreen world, there are two types of sunscreens, organic and inorganic. In this sense, the meaning of organic sunscreen is in reference to chemistry and the use of carbon-based chemicals called photostabilizers (like oxybenzone, avobenzone, octanoate, and homosalate) to block the UV radiation from entering our skin cells. While the goal is noble, the chemicals used to accomplish the task are harmful to our health and the health of the environment and marine life. One of the main ingredients, oxybenzone, has been known to disrupt endocrine function by mimicking estrogen in the body, disrupting reproductive function in both sexes. Others may be carcinogenic (cancer-causing). Inorganic sunscreen filters, on the other hand, work by reflecting and scattering the radiation. They are not as easily absorbed and therefore are known to be much less toxic to your body. The two main ingredients, zinc oxide and titanium dioxide, are used in natural sunscreens and offer safer alternatives than their chemical-filled counterparts. However, they often leave white chalky residue on your face. Zinc oxide is believed to be the most effective and safest mineral UV filter. Suggestions: Some popular natural sunscreen brands include MyChelle, Annmarie, Beauty Counter, Goddess Garden, and Badger.

Self-Tanners. If you must...look for a natural sugar beet dihydroxyacetone (DHA) without parabens, sulfates, or other harmful preservatives such as Naru Organics, Whish, Beauty by Earth, Chocolate Sun, Mine, etc.

Lip Balms. Ditch the Chap Stick for Burt's Bees, Dr. Bronner's, Badger, Alba Botanica, etc.

Talc. Talc is an ingredient that is extracted from rock deposits to produce talcum powder for use many cosmetics, from baby powder to blush. Talc has been found to contain asbestos and can be dangerous if inhaled or absorbed into the skin. Manufacturing companies transform it into a soft, fine talcum powder. Despite the large class action lawsuits and ongoing FDA studies, it is still widely used in products today. Johnson & Johnson stopped selling baby powder containing talc in North America in 2020 after agreeing to the payment of over 9 billion dollars in settlement damages. In addition, they have recently discontinued global use of talc and have replaced it with a cornstarch-based baby powder formula.

Replace any cosmetics containing talc. If dusting powder containing talc is part of your daily regimen for you or your baby, replace it with brands such as Burt's Bees, Era Organics, California Baby, Hello Bello, or Beachcomber.

Eye Drops. Ditch the Visine and Clear Eyes and go for homeopathic or preservative-free brands. Health food stores are good sources as they have done preliminary research for us.

Plastic Water Bottles. It is no secret that plastic bottles contain numerous harmful chemicals, although the real issue arises when our water bottles sit in the hot car or sun and leach into the water we will be drinking. The leaching process may begin in transport before they hit the market shelves. You may have noticed grocery stores displaying cases of bottled water outside the store baking in the hot sun. Make it a habit to store filtered water in a non-toxic bottle or container when you are out. In addition, hot foods should be stored in glass containers instead of plastic.

Household Products. Some of the most harmful products that touch our skin and that we breathe through our lungs come from our everyday household products. Although we can't live in a bubble and avoid toxins altogether, we can decrease the amount of toxins we come in contact with by replacing our toxic household cleansers.

Air Fresheners. Commercial air fresheners, including candles containing VOCs, contain several toxic chemicals. They cause air pollution in the home and are harmful to people and pets. One simple action to improve the air quality in your home is to switch from conventional air fresheners to healthier options. Suggestions: Non-Aerosol brands containing pure essential oils. Air Scense is a good one for bathroom use. Consider aromatherapy diffusers using quality essential oils, and natural candles made with organic soy, beeswax, or palm wax. Natural candles use essential oils and other natural ingredients for fragrance. For reed diffusers and room mists, check out rareESSENCE Aromatherapy.

Laundry Detergents. Although your clothes might smell as fresh as a summer breeze, the reality is that many commercial laundry detergents contain harmful chemicals that can lead to negative health effects and seep into the bloodstream from the residual left on your clothing and sheets. Research links many of these chemicals to contact dermatitis, hormone imbalance, endocrine disruption, respiratory dysfunction, and even cancer. These chemicals also negatively affect our environment.

Suggestions: ECOS Plant Powered Laundry Detergent, Zum Laundry Soap by Indigo Wild, Charlie's Soap Laundry Powder (they also carry Oxygen Bleach, a safe, non-chlorine bleach).

Aerosols. Many household products come in an aerosol can, such as air fresheners, furniture polish, hair spray, and deodorants. When aerosols are sprayed, a cloud of chemicals in a fine mist is released into the air, sometimes using highly flammable butane. The aerosol you breathe in enters your bloodstream and may cause issues such as headaches, damage to the central nervous system, liver and kidney dysfunction, asthma, and has even been linked with an increased risk of cancer. They can also damage the lungs and cause skin, eye, and throat irritation. Suggestions: Seek products that are in pump spray bottles.

All-Purpose Cleaners. All-purpose cleaners are supposed to make cleaning easier since you can use them on practically any surface in your house. Unfortunately, they can contain an assortment of toxic chemicals including *fragrance* (a catch-all phrase that can hide up to 100 undisclosed ingredients). Suggestions: Although many health-conscious people like to make their own with vinegar, I'm not a fan. All-purpose cleaners from essential oil companies are a nice choice and smell much better. Some nice healthier alternatives are Charlie's Professional, ECOS, biokleen, Dr. Bronner's, Seventh Generation, and Bon Ami Powder Cleanser.

Floor Cleaning Products. For hardwood, vinyl, and stone, try Naturally It's Clean Floor Enzyme Floor Cleaner, biokleen Bac-out Multi-Surface Floor Cleaner, Aunt Fannie's, Norwex cleaning products, and Shark Steam Mop (cleans with just water). Using a vacuum with HEPA filter will trap 99.97% of the dust inside your vacuum, keeping it out of the air you breathe.

Glass Cleaners. Let the chemical-based ones go! Less toxic brands include Better Life Natural Streak Free, Everspring, biokleen Glass Cleaner, ECOS, Simple Green Naturals, Homesolv, Greenshield Organic, and Athos.

Indoor Air. The American College of Allergists says that 50% of illnesses are caused or worsened by polluted indoor air. Air purification systems can be added to your HVAC system. REME-HALO offers an in-home filtration system to eliminate viruses, bacteria, mold spores, and chemical toxins. Alternatively, look into a good stand-alone air filter.

Cookware. The ongoing battle to remove Teflon due to the chemical known as polytetrafluoroethylene (PTFE), and its proven health hazards of this chemical leaching into cooked foods and into our bloodstreams, resulted in DuPont, 3M and other companies producing a "safer" alternative. Unfortunately, this replacement, which goes by the name of GenX, has proven to be just as harmful as its predecessor. It is imperative that we discard any unhealthy non-stick containing PTFE, PFOA, or anything labeled as nonstick. The best alternatives in order of preference are ceramic (which is nonstick), cast iron, carbon steel, and stainless steel. Some favorite brands include: Le Creuset (enameled cast iron), Caraway (ceramic-coated aluminum), Our Place (ceramic-coated aluminum), Scanpan (ceramic-titanium finish), and Misen (carbon steel), to name a few.

Dry Cleaning. Conventional cleaners submerge garments in Perchloroethylene (Perc), a solvent with a sweet, ether-like odor, to remove dirt and soil and dissolve greases, oils, and waxes without water. This toxic chemical has been found to cause adverse health effects in some individuals if absorbed into the skin from the garment, as well as an air pollutant. Eco-friendly green dry cleaners, although more expensive, may be a better option. Most of these cleaners utilize the GreenEarth® cleaning method to replace perc. GreenEarth® is liquified sand. It is also known as $SiO2$. It works as a solvent known as siloxane. Once GreenEarth® is thrown away, then it breaks into sand, $CO2$, and water.

Tap Water. Neither you nor your pets should ever drink tap water. Water filters come in a variety of different prices and types and should be used by all households. This topic will be discussed in more detail in the Hydrate chapter.

***

This list can go on and on, but we have covered some of the basics. For those wanting to dig further down this rabbit hole, more information on toxins within the household can be learned from a documentary titled *Stink,* which can be found on Netflix. I also highly recommend the Live Longer video by the Live Better Group found on www.thelivebettergroup.com/25ways.

Chapter 5
EMFs & Radiation

EMFs (electromagnetic frequencies) and radiation. Often when my clients get tested because they are suffering from lack of energy or chronic fatigue, insomnia or ill health, at least one component of either radiation or EMFs shows up as the culprit. Regardless of whether you believe you are experiencing symptoms from EMFs, they are still affecting us on a cellular level and contribute to disease.

It is not uncommon for people to be electro-sensitive and experience an allergic reaction to cell phones, cordless phones, Wi-Fi routers, Bluetooth gadgets, or even cell phone towers near your home or office without even knowing the culprit. And now that the new 5G (and above) cellular networks and tens of thousands of satellites are being rolled out, more people are feeling a constant zapping sensation and experiencing symptoms like fatigue, sleep disturbances, including insomnia, headaches, migraines, heart palpitations, depression or mood disorders, brain fog, dizziness, irritability, restlessness, anxiety, nausea, and skin problems including burning and tingling.

When most people think about radiation exposure, imaging devices for X-rays and CT scans come to mind. However, our power lines, cellphones, microwaves, Wi-Fi routers, wireless devices, computer screens, televisions, and other appliances send out a stream of invisible energy waves. Electromagnetic frequencies (EMFs) are produced anywhere electricity is used, including at home and in the workplace. Again, as with other household toxins, exposure to only one item or appliance may not be an issue. However, the cumulative exposure from multiple sources can bombard our cells. Throughout the years, there has been ongoing disagreement in scientific literature over whether EMFs pose a danger to human health and, if so, how much. The International Agency for Research on Cancer (IARC) has classified certain types of EMFs as carcinogenic. Electronic products like cell phones, smart devices, and tablets operate in these fields. Each source is classified into varying degrees of danger and emits some radiation output to some degree.

Top environmental medicine doctors are seeing increasing numbers of people develop what they are labeling as electro-sensitivity, a disorder where one becomes allergic to these electromagnetic waves. However, just because one does not *feel* the effects, our cells are nevertheless receiving them, which could very well be another silent killer in our midst. There is not a lot we can do about the rollout of new technology, but there are things we can do to mitigate the damage once we are aware of what they are.

The following tips and guidelines of things to avoid, limit, or replace, help to limit exposure as every small change matters.

Electric Blankets. Electric blankets emit low-frequency electromagnetic fields (ELFs) when plugged in and especially when turned on. These EMFs can disrupt the body's natural bioelectric balance, which is finely tuned to very subtle electrical signals. They can potentially interfere with melatonin production and the body's circadian rhythm if used during sleep. In addition, they can create oxidative stress and low-level inflammation in sensitive individuals or those already EMF-reactive. If you must use an electric blanket, use it only to preheat the bed and turn it off before sleeping. This minimizes EMF exposure and prevents overheating, allowing your body's natural temperature rhythms and biofield to restore balance during rest.

Cell Phones. If you keep your phone in your bedroom while sleeping, place it in airplane mode nightly. The alarm setting will still work. Preferably, turn the phone off altogether. If unable to turn the phone off, place it across the room instead of on the nightstand.

Baby Monitors. Place them across the rooms (away from the baby's and your head) to limit EMF exposure.

Smart Meters. Start meters are not so smart. They are making households sick. Either purchase a faraday cage smart meter cover (found on Amazon) or have it removed. For more information, visit www.takebackyourpower.net.

Microwaves. Irradiating your food is not the only thing that is getting fried. As mentioned earlier, ditch the microwave. If you occasionally must use it, at the very least, do not stand peering into it while your food cooks. Get as far away from it as possible so that the radiation it is emitting is only going into your food and not into you as well.

The Internet of Things. If you can live without a smart home that does everything for you at the drop of a command, opt out.

Metal-Framed Glasses. Metal frames, as conductors of energy, can reflect and refocus wireless radiation, leading to higher localized absorption into the body. In fact, one study found that wearing metal-framed glasses can increase radiation exposure in those areas by up to tenfold (according to a 2020 electromagnetic safety study). For those who are energy-sensitive or simply wish to minimize exposure, non-metal frames made of wood, plastic, or natural fibers can help reduce electromagnetic absorption and better support cellular health.

Wireless Phone Chargers. Replace them with wired chargers. They are much safer and much more efficient.

Bluetooth Headsets. Replace with a simple set of earphones. Or better yet, use speaker mode and keep your phone as far away from your body as possible. Bluetooth is a mini-Wi-Fi signal relating to all the problems that we are trying to avoid.

Medical Imaging. There are times when medical imaging cannot be avoided. Taking chlorella tablets before and after the procedure can help your body eliminate residual radiation. Routine checkups such as mammograms also emit radiation, so consider utilizing thermography instead. This technology is said to detect breast cancer years earlier than traditional imaging—without the cancer-causing radiation or false positives. Note that thermography is typically not covered by medical insurance.

Radiation from Air Travel. Although the TSA has the right to deny your request, always ask for a pat-down instead of entering the full-body scanner. The millimeter-wave technology used in the scanners to disclose weapons hidden under clothing penetrates the body with radiation. Although the manufacturer states that the radiation received is non-ionizing, (meaning it does not have enough energy to damage DNA directly) and is not known to be genotoxic, natural medical doctors have claimed it is equivalent to having 10 CT scans. People who travel frequently should always try to petition for a pat-down. Occasional travelers may be fine, while others may experience dizziness or fatigue for hours to days. EMFs are throughout the airport as well as on your flight, so for the sake of your health, take extra chlorella on travel days and wear a personal protection shield such as shungite jewelry and Lambs protective clothing or Qi Me from Synergy Science, or other similar devices.

5G Towers and Power Lines. At the time of this writing, we are still on 5G. Before long, we will be going to 6G and beyond. When purchasing a home or spending 8 hours or more in the workplace, make sure you are within a safe distance of these environmental hazards. It is documented that you should reside at least 700 feet from high-voltage power lines, although the farther the better. It is a good practice to place Lemurian Plugs throughout your home (https://www.thelemurianplug.com). To check to see how close you are to any 5G towers, visit: www.antennasearch.com and enter your zip code.

This concludes the portion of items that we should remove from our diet, home, and environment. Thank you for bearing with this information. I know these are grim topics, but, for the sake of our health, they need to be covered. Although it's not conclusive by any means, it is a comprehensive start to where we need to be. A conscious effort to improve along these lines will significantly benefit our health.

Chapter 6
Gut Health

"All Disease Starts in the Gut" – Hippocrates

The Gut as the Center of Immunity

The importance of gut health cannot be stressed enough. Nearly 70–80% of the body's immune system resides in the gut, particularly within the intestinal lining and the trillions of microbes that call it home. This makes the gut more than a digestive organ—it is a command center for immunity, constantly interacting with the outside world through the food, microbes, and environmental particles we ingest. The gut is responsible for our protection through three different methods:

- Gut-Associated Lymphoid Tissue (GALT): These are specialized immune cells that line the gut wall, acting as sentinels that recognize and neutralize invaders while allowing nutrients and friendly microbes to pass.

- The Microbiome: A diverse colony of bacteria, fungi, and other microbes help train the immune system to distinguish between friend and foe. Beneficial bacteria also outcompete pathogens, preventing infections from taking hold.

- The Gut Barrier: The intestinal lining serves as a selective filter—absorbing nutrients while blocking toxins and pathogens. When this barrier is strong, the entire body benefits.

In many ancient traditions, the gut was regarded as the body's true center of strength and vitality—and modern science now beautifully echoes that wisdom. When we care for the gut, we're not just improving digestion; we're nurturing the foundation of immunity, energy, and emotional balance. A healthy gut allows us to do more than resist disease—it empowers us to thrive physically, mentally, and spiritually. With strong digestive health, the immune system becomes more resilient, shielding us from colds, flu viruses, chronic inflammation, and even autoimmune flare-ups. Energy and mood stabilize as inflammation subsides, allowing the brain to receive steady signals of wellbeing. Nutrients such as B12, vitamin K, and essential minerals like magnesium are absorbed more efficiently, fueling every cell with vitality. A balanced gut microbiome also supports healthy weight and metabolism by regulating appetite and blood sugar levels. Even our outer radiance reflects our inner harmony—clearer skin and a youthful glow are natural byproducts of reduced systemic inflammation and a thriving digestive ecosystem.

The Gut is so Much More Than Digestion. When people talk about the "gut," they often think only of the stomach. But the gut is a vast and intricate system that begins at the mouth and ends at the rectum, working tirelessly to digest, absorb, and protect. It includes:

- **Mouth and Esophagus**: the entryway for food, beginning digestion with enzymes in the saliva.

- **Stomach**: the acidic chamber that breaks food into smaller particles.

- **Small Intestine:** where most nutrient absorption occurs with the help of digestive enzymes and bile.

- **Large Intestine (Colon)**: the home of trillions of microbes that ferment fiber, produce vitamins, and regulate immunity.

- **Liver, Gallbladder, and Pancreas**: accessory organs that produce bile, enzymes, and hormones, orchestrating smooth digestion.

Together, these organs form not just a digestive system but an ecosystem—a living environment where food, microbes, and human cells interact to shape health on every level. Today with all the toxins and environmental factors, we are becoming sicker than ever, and gut health is suffering. One may wonder how the gut falls out of balance in the first place. Quite simply, the gut thrives on harmony, but modern lifestyles often disturb its delicate ecosystem. Some of the most common disruptors include:

- **Poor Diet**: Excess sugar, refined carbs, and processed foods feed harmful bacteria while starving beneficial microbes.

- **Antibiotics & Prescription Medications**: Although they may be necessary, they come with side effects. Antibiotics and common drugs like NSAIDs can strip away the protective microbiome and damage the gut lining.

- **Chronic Stress**: Stress hormones reduce blood flow to the digestive tract, alter motility, and weaken the gut-brain connection.

- **Toxins and Environmental Factors**: Pesticides, heavy metals, alcohol, and chemicals compromise gut barrier integrity.

- **Sedentary Lifestyle**: Lack of movement slows digestion and can disrupt microbial diversity.

Our gut is home to a vast inner ecosystem known as the microbiome, a community of trillions of bacteria, viruses, fungi, and other microorganisms. In fact, the gut contains more microbial cells than the entire human body has human cells. These tiny residents are not intruders; they are partners in health, performing essential roles such as:

Digesting Fiber: Beneficial bacteria ferment fibers we cannot digest, producing short-chain fatty acids (SCFAs) that nourish the colon lining and reduce inflammation.

Producing Nutrients: Some gut microbes make vitamins such as vitamin K and certain B vitamins.

Training Immunity: The microbiome teaches the immune system how to distinguish intruders from allies

Regulating Mood: By producing neurotransmitters (serotonin, dopamine, GABA), gut bacteria influence the gut-brain connection and emotional wellbeing.

When this microbial garden is diverse and balanced, it forms a protective shield against disease and fosters resilience. But what happens when the bad microbes overpopulate the good ones, and how does the gut fall out of balance in the first place?

Dysbiosis: When the Bad Outnumber the Good. The gut microbiome is like a rainforest: every species contributes to the overall balance. But modern lifestyles—poor diet, antibiotics, toxins, chronic stress—can disrupt this balance, leading to dysbiosis (an imbalance between beneficial and harmful microbes). This is what happens when the body is in dysbiosis.

Overgrowth of Harmful Bacteria: "Bad" bacteria or yeast species multiply, producing toxins, gas, and inflammatory compounds.

Damage to the Gut Lining: Harmful microbes erode the mucosal barrier, making the intestine more permeable, causing leaky gut.

Immune System Overactivation: When sensing invaders, the immune system goes into constant defense mode, fueling inflammation.

Nutrient Deficiency: With less room for beneficial bacteria, production of vitamins and absorption of minerals declines.

Digestive Symptoms: Bloating, diarrhea, constipation, and abdominal pain often follow.

Systemic Effects: Dysbiosis has been linked not only to digestive disorders but also to skin conditions, autoimmune disease, depression, and metabolic disorders.

Restoring Balance

Just as weeds can overtake a neglected garden, harmful microbes thrive when the inner terrain weakens. Healing requires:

Feeding the Good: Fiber-rich vegetables, legumes, seeds, and resistant starches act as *prebiotics* that nourish beneficial bacteria.

Repopulating with Allies: Probiotics and fermented foods introduce diverse, health-promoting strains.

Creating Hostile Conditions for Harmful Microbes – Reducing sugar, alcohol, and processed foods weakens "bad" bacteria and yeast.

Reinforcing the Gut Barrier – Nutrients like L-glutamine, zinc, and omega-3s repair the intestinal lining, supporting microbial balance.

Common Gut Disorders. Imbalances can manifest in a wide spectrum of diseases:

Irritable Bowel Syndrome (IBS) – Functional disorder linked to dysbiosis, stress, and food sensitivities. Symptoms include bloating, cramping, and irregular bowel movements.

Inflammatory Bowel Disease (IBD) – Includes Crohn's disease and ulcerative colitis, autoimmune-driven inflammation damaging the intestinal lining.

Celiac Disease – An autoimmune condition triggered by gluten, leading to intestinal damage and nutrient malabsorption.

Small Intestinal Bacterial Overgrowth (SIBO) – Overgrowth of bacteria in the small intestine causes bloating, gas, and malabsorption.

Leaky Gut Syndrome – Increased intestinal permeability linked to allergies, autoimmunity, and chronic inflammation.

GERD (Acid Reflux): Acid reflux occurs when stomach acid flows back into the esophagus, causing burning, discomfort, or regurgitation. Acid reflux can also be experienced by people with a hiatal hernia, a condition where part of the stomach pushes upward through the diaphragm into the chest cavity, preventing acid from escaping.

Diarrhea: Occasional diarrhea is often due to infections, food intolerances, or sudden changes in diet. It will usually resolve quickly once the trigger is gone. Chronic diarrhea is a red flag for deeper imbalances like inflammatory bowel disease, celiac disease, food allergies, or gut dysbiosis, infections (bacterial, viral, parasitic), medications or certain supplements, or stress and anxiety (fight-or-flight mode speeds motility).

Constipation: Constipation occurs when bowel movements become infrequent, difficult, or incomplete. While many dismiss it as a minor inconvenience, chronic constipation is a signal from the gut that balance has been disrupted. The three types are 1) Slow-transit **is** where the colon muscles move too slowly, causing stool to remain in the intestine for too long and become hard and dry; 2) Outlet is where the stool reaches the rectum, but the muscles needed for elimination don't coordinate properly, making it difficult to pass, and 3) Secondary Constipation is triggered by external factors such as medications, low thyroid function, dehydration, or even travel and disrupted routines. Several factors may converge to slow the natural rhythm of the gut such as lack of fiber and whole foods in the diet, insufficient hydration, sedentary lifestyle, disruption of the gut microbiome, often from antibiotics, processed foods, or stress, or an emotional component of "holding on," as unresolved tension and perfectionism can manifest physically.

Regular and Healthy Bowel Movements. Many people don't realize that regular elimination is one of the body's primary detox systems. When bowel movements are delayed or irregular, waste lingers in the body, which can affect everything from energy to immunity. Every day, our bodies process not only food but also toxins, hormones, and byproducts of metabolism. When stools don't move regularly, these substances can be reabsorbed into the bloodstream, increasing the toxic burden. Furthermore, excess hormones like estrogen are excreted through the stool. If elimination slows down, hormones can recirculate, leading to hormone imbalances such as PMS, mood swings, or skin issues. I understand that all this talk about stools may constitute too much information (TMI) for some, but rest assured, it's very important for our health to understand what the consequences may be so appropriate changes can be made.

The Bristol Stool Chart is used by medical professionals to explain the seven types of elimination and the healthy ones we should strive for.

BRISTOL STOOL CHART

Type 1	Separate hard lumps, like nuts
Type 2	Sausage-shaped but lumpy
Type 3	Like a sausage but with cracks on the surface
Type 4	Like a sausage or snake, smooth and soft
Type 5	Soft blobs with clear-cut edges
Type 6	Fluffy pieces with ragged edges mushy stool
Type 7	Watery, no solid pieces, entirely liquid

Form and Shape: **Type 1:** Separate hard lumps, like nuts indicate constipation, dehydration, and slow transit. **Type 2:** Sausage-shaped but lumpy **is s**till a sign of constipation; stool is moving but too slowly. **Type 3:**

Like a sausage but with cracks on the surface is a near-ideal stool that is comfortable to pass, showing good balance of fiber and hydration. **Type 4:** Like a sausage or snake, smooth and soft is considered *the healthiest stool*. This is what we should strive for—easy to pass, formed, and well-hydrated. **Type 5:** Soft blobs with clear-cut edges are a sign of rapid transit; may occur after stress, mild food sensitivities, or eating a lot of fruit/fiber. **Type 6:** Fluffy pieces with ragged edges, mushy stool suggest diarrhea, inflammation, or imbalance in the gut microbiome. **Type 7:** Watery, no solid pieces, entirely liquid indicate diarrhea, often due to infection, food poisoning, or severe imbalance.

Color: Brown is normal (thanks to bile). Very pale, black, or red stools may signal issues and should be checked medically.

Ease of Elimination: Stools should pass without straining, urgency, or pain. Healthy elimination feels complete and effortless.

Frequency: Once to twice per day is considered healthy. Some individuals go three times per day, others every other day—what matters most is consistency, comfort, and ease.

The Gut-Brain Connection: Our Second Brain. You've probably heard the phrase "follow your gut." Science shows there's truth in this wisdom. The gut doesn't just digest food—it also produces neurotransmitters and sends signals that shape our mood and decision-making. Also, when the gut is balanced, those intuitive nudges are clearer, calmer, and more trustworthy. This is another example of how everything within our body is connected.

The communication system between the gut (the gastrointestinal tract) and brain (the central nervous system) is referred to as the gut-brain axis. It's a complex, dynamic network that links digestion, mood, depression and anxiety, sleep, learning, memory, hormones, immune function, and even behavior. They're connected both physically and biochemically in a number of different ways. They may even influence each other's health. Modern science confirms what ancient healing traditions have long taught: the gut and brain are intimately linked. The gut is sometimes called the "second brain" because of the enteric nervous system—a vast network of over 100 million nerve cells embedded in the intestinal walls communicating with the brain. Let's break it down for better understanding.

Neural Pathways and the Vagus Nerve. The vagus nerve is the main "superhighway" connecting the gut and the brain. Signals about digestion, satiety, inflammation, and discomfort travel from the gut lining to the brain, and in return the brain sends signals that can affect gut motility, secretion, and sensitivity. For example, stress can trigger stomach cramps, while a calm mind can ease digestion.

Microbiome Influence. As previously discussed, trillions of bacteria, fungi, and other microbes in the gut produce neuroactive compounds (like serotonin, dopamine, and GABA) that influence mood, cognition, and stress resilience. About 90–95% of the body's serotonin is actually produced in the gut. A balanced microbiome helps regulate inflammation and supports neurotransmitter production, while dysbiosis (imbalance) can contribute to anxiety, depression, or digestive disorders.

Immune System & Inflammation. In recapping the immune system, around 70% – 80% of the immune system resides in the gut. The gut lining and microbiota interact with immune cells, releasing cytokines (messenger molecules) that can affect the brain's inflammatory status. Chronic gut inflammation is linked to conditions like depression, brain fog, and neurodegenerative diseases.

Hormonal & Endocrine Signals. The gut produces hormones such as ghrelin (hunger hormone), leptin (satiety), and cortisol regulators that influence appetite, metabolism, and stress. These hormones travel through the bloodstream and signal the brain about the body's energy and nutritional status.

Psychological & Emotional Feedback. Emotions such as stress, anxiety, and joy directly influence gut function through the autonomic nervous system. That's why people use phrases like "butterflies in your stomach" or "gut feeling."

Gut Bacteria and Emotional Health. Being that the gut biome affects emotional health (depression, stress, anxiety) and cognitive functioning (memory, attention, aging); it would only make sense that improving gut bacteria may be an excellent place to start on any healing journey. The diet and lifestyle suggestions in Part One, along with adding a probiotic and a prebiotic may greatly improve depression and anxiety. Although not a "quick fix" over the course of a few weeks, relief may be noticed in a big way. It takes time but in comparison, starting a course of antidepressants (that ironically have a side effect of further messing up the gut microbiome) also takes this long to kick in so patience is key. It is recommended to consult with a doctor before starting or going off any type of medication.

Probiotics and Prebiotics: Adding Good Bacteria to Improve Gut Health

Probiotics. There are varieties of probiotic supplements that contain live (good) bacteria to support gut health. Probiotics *add* good bacteria whereas prebiotics are nondigestible fibers that are fermented by your gut bacteria that *feed* the good bacteria that's already there. However, not all probiotics are created equal. Without knowing, many people search Amazon for a general, multi-strain probiotic and take it without researching the benefits of all the different types. Different types of strains can be quite specialized for different needs and may be more beneficial than a generic choice. Often trial and error is needed if the first one isn't helping the symptoms for which it is being used.

For example, specialized probiotics that affect the brain are often referred to as psychobiotics. Fructo-oligosaccharides (FOS) and galacto-oligosaccharides (GOS): have been found to mitigate depressive symptoms and are linked to lower cortisol and improved emotional processing.

Here's a structured overview of common probiotic types, their strains, and the gut-related symptoms or conditions they are most often associated with.

Lactobacillus species: These are some of the most studied probiotics and are naturally found in the small intestine and fermented foods.

- **Lactobacillus acidophilus:** Helps with: lactose intolerance, diarrhea (including antibiotic-associated), mild IBS, candida overgrowth.

- **Lactobacillus rhamnosus GG (LGG):** Helps with: acute infectious diarrhea, traveler's diarrhea, antibiotic-associated diarrhea, eczema in children.

- **Lactobacillus plantarum:** Helps with: IBS bloating and pain, ulcerative colitis, improving gut lining integrity ("leaky gut").

- **Lactobacillus casei:** Helps with: constipation, diarrhea prevention, enhancing immune response.

- **Lactobacillus reuteri:** Helps with: colic in infants, gut motility issues, oral health, and some evidence for reducing *Helicobacter pylori* infection.

Bifidobacterium species: Primarily reside in the colon and are especially important in infants and overall colon health.

- **Bifidobacterium bifidum:** Helps with: diarrhea, IBS, improving overall digestion and nutrient absorption.

- **Bifidobacterium longum:** Helps with: reducing inflammation, improving IBS symptoms, lactose intolerance, and anxiety linked to gut-brain axis.

- **Bifidobacterium breve:** Helps with constipation, skin issues (eczema), reducing weight gain in children at risk of obesity.

- **Bifidobacterium infantis (35624 strain):** Helps with: IBS symptoms (pain, bloating, gas), immune regulation, reducing gut inflammation.

Saccharomyces boulardii (a probiotic yeast): Helps with: antibiotic-associated diarrhea, traveler's diarrhea, *Clostridium difficile* recurrence prevention, IBS-D (diarrhea-predominant IBS).

Streptococcus thermophilus: Helps with: lactose digestion, diarrhea prevention, and supporting beneficial gut bacteria balance.

Spore-forming / Soil-based probiotics (Bacillus species): These strains survive stomach acid well and are more resilient.

- **Bacillus coagulans:** Helps with: IBS symptoms, constipation, diarrhea, immune modulation.

- **Bacillus subtilis:** Helps with: improving digestion, enhancing gut microbiome diversity, reducing bloating.

Multi-strain blends: Many commercial probiotics combine Lactobacillus + Bifidobacterium + sometimes Saccharomyces or Bacillus. These blends often target: IBS (both diarrhea and constipation types), Leaky gut and inflammation, Recovery after antibiotics, and General digestive support

Main Types of Prebiotics

Prebiotics are specialized plant fibers that nourish the beneficial bacteria already living in your gut. Unlike probiotics (which are live bacteria), prebiotics are non-digestible food components in the form of certain fibers and resistant starches that pass through the digestive system and serve

PROBIOTICS AND GUT HEALTH

PROBIOTIC TYPE	HELPS WITH
Lactobacillus species Lactobacillus acidophilus Lactobacillus rhamnesus GG Lactobacillus plantarum Lactobacillus casei Lactobaciilus reuteri	Lactose intolerance Diarrhea (including antibiotic-antidiatc-aesciated) Mild IBS, candida overgrowth Acute infectious diarrhea Traveler's diarrhea Antibiotic associated diarrhea Eczema in children
Bifidobacterium species Bifidobacterium bifidum Bifidobacterium longum Bifidobacterium breze Bifidobacterium infantis	IBS bloating and pain Ulcerative colitis Improving gut linng integrity (leaky gut)
Saccharomyces boulardii Bacillus coagulans Bacillus subtilis	Constipation Diarrhea prevention Enhancing immune: resolution
Streptococcus thermphil- Lactose digestion Diarrhea prevention Supporting beneficial gut bacteria balance	Constipation, skin issues (eczem) Reducing weight gain in children a risk of obesity
	IBS symptom, bin lesues, lactesal Reducing gut imflammation
Spore-forming/ Soil-based (*Bacillus species*)	IBS (both diarrhea a constipation) Leaky gut and inflammation Recovery after antibiotics
Multi-strain blends	

as food for gut microbes. Normally a balanced diet rich in plant-based whole foods usually provides enough prebiotics without supplementation. But targeted prebiotic powders (like inulin or GOS) are available if extra support is needed. Here's a breakdown:

- **Fructooligosaccharides (FOS):** Found in bananas, onions, garlic, leeks, asparagus, chicory root. Its function is to promote *Bifidobacteria* growth and help balance gut flora.

- **Galactooligosaccharides (GOS):** Found in legumes (beans, lentils, chickpeas), some dairy products. Function: enhance both *Bifidobacteria* and *Lactobacilli* populations.

- **Inulin:** Found in chicory root, Jerusalem artichoke, dandelion greens, garlic, onions. Its function improves calcium absorption, supports digestive health, and boosts satiety.

- **Resistant Starch:** Found in cooked-and-cooled potatoes and rice, green bananas, oats, legumes. It ferments in the large intestine, producing short-chain fatty acids (SCFAs) like butyrate, which nourish colon cells.

- **Beta-glucans:** Found in: oats, barley, and mushrooms. They function to support immune function and help regulate cholesterol and blood sugar.

- **Pectins:** Found in apples, citrus fruits, and carrots. Pectins create a gel-forming fiber that supports digestion and may lower cholesterol.

Where to begin?

As we have discussed, the gut is related to most of our health issues. If you have a healthy gut with healthy elimination, can eat most foods without consequences, and have no stomach upset or symptoms, excellent! Keep doing what you are doing.

If you have been diagnosed with any of the following conditions: IBS, IBD, leaky gut, diverticulitis, celiac disease, SIBO, or GERD, or are experiencing symptoms such as chronic bloating, belching, painful gas, indigestion, heartburn, acid reflux, gout, diarrhea, constipation, skin conditions (acne, eczema, rosacea), cognitive decline, brain fog, trouble concentrating, emotional issues (depression, anxiety, mood changes), insomnia, fatigue, headaches or migraines, sugar cravings, unexplained weight gain, inflammation, frequent colds or weakened immunity, the GUT is the first place to start. The chances are very high that something in your diet and an imbalance in your gut is taking place. Because gut health is complicated, it may feel overwhelming knowing where to begin. It is always best to work with a holistic health practitioner that specializes in gut health to speed along your process.

- **Food Sensitivity Testing**: One often wonders...what comes first the chicken or the egg. Do harmful foods cause gut disturbances or does an unhealthy gut cause food sensitivity? In some cases, it can be both. We will want to eliminate all the foods that are currently triggering health issues. Blood tests and kinesiology are good; however, I recommend bioenergetic testing (explained in Section Three) as it will not only list all the individual food culprits, but it will also identify phenolic sensitivities which are so important. Phenolics are a large group of natural compounds found in plants, especially in fruits, vegetables, teas, herbs, and spices. They act as antioxidants and give foods much of their color, flavor, and aroma. Examples include flavonoids, tannins, and salicylates. Some people are not necessarily sensitive to the food itself, but to the phenolic compounds within it. For instance: A person might tolerate apples in general but react to the salicylates (a type of phenolic) they contain. Symptoms of phenolic sensitivity can include headaches, skin rashes, asthma-like reactions, cognitive issues, anxiety, or digestive upset. This differs from a classic "food allergy," which involves the immune system reacting to proteins in a food. Instead, phenolic sensitivity is more about how the body metabolizes and detoxifies these plant compounds (often linked to enzyme pathways like sulfation), which is important to know. Bioenergetic testing will also identify any types of non-food disturbances that may be causing issues within the gut such as parasites or other protozoa, candida overgrowth, mycotoxins, etc., which is helpful for knowing what to treat.

- **Incorporate a Whole Foods Diet:** After learning your food sensitivities, begin with your healthy diet (minus the foods you will want to avoid for now). Remove all fast foods, packaged/processed foods, and inflammatory foods from your diet (fried foods, sugar, refined carbohydrates, trans fats & hydrogenated oils, vegetable oils, and alcohol).

- **Restoring Gut Balance:** Healing the gut requires a multi-layered approach—scientific, nutritional, and holistic. Many practitioners use the "4R" framework that includes:

    ○ **Remove** – Identify and eliminate irritants (processed foods, allergens, alcohol, excess caffeine).

- **Replace** – Support digestion with enzymes, stomach acid, and bile salts if needed.

- **Reinoculate** – Restore microbiome balance with probiotics, prebiotics, and fermented foods.

- **Repair** – Heal the gut lining with nutrients such as L-glutamine, zinc, omega-3s, collagen, and soothing herbs like slippery elm and aloe vera.

Enhancing Food Absorption: Nourishing from the Inside Out. You may have heard the *phrase "You are not what you eat — you are what you absorb."* While the types of food we consume matters, how well we assimilate it matters even more. Without proper absorption, even the most vibrant foods can't deliver their healing potential. In other words, we can eat the cleanest, most nutrient-dense foods in the world, but if our bodies can't absorb them properly, those nutrients never reach the cells where healing and energy truly happen. Food absorption is the bridge between eating and nourishment — the process that transforms what we consume into the raw materials for vitality, repair, and radiance. Factors That Inhibit Absorption

Certain habits and substances can reduce your ability to absorb nutrients such as eating under stress or rushing meals, overuse of antibiotics or antacids, high alcohol, caffeine, or sugar intake, chronic inflammation or food sensitivities, or nutrient competition (e.g., calcium and iron competing for absorption sites). Awareness of these obstacles allows you to make small, mindful changes that dramatically improve nutrient assimilation.

The Journey of Digestion and Absorption. Absorption begins long before food reaches the intestines. In fact, it starts in the mouth, where chewing activates enzymes in saliva that begin breaking down carbohydrates. As food moves to the stomach, gastric acid and enzymes continue the process, preparing nutrients for entry into the small intestine, which is the primary site of absorption.

Within the small intestine, millions of microscopic projections called villi and microvilli line the intestinal walls. These finger-like structures increase the surface area for nutrient absorption, allowing vitamins, minerals, amino acids, and fatty acids to pass into the bloodstream.

The liver and gallbladder also play vital supporting roles: bile helps emulsify fats, making them easier to digest and absorb, while the liver filters and processes nutrients before sending them throughout the body. Meanwhile, your gut microbiome with trillions of beneficial bacteria helps break down fiber, produce B-vitamins, and even support the absorption of minerals like magnesium and calcium.

When absorption is compromised, even healthy eating can leave you undernourished. Be on the lookout for these signals: persistent bloating or gas, undigested food in stool, fatigue or brain fog, brittle nails or thinning hair, dry skin or dull complexion, or nutrient deficiencies (especially iron, B12, or vitamin D). These symptoms often point to an imbalance in the gut lining or a disrupted microbiome — both of which can be repaired with care and awareness.

Optimizing food absorption isn't about eating more — it's about eating *wisely* and creating the right internal conditions for digestion to thrive. Factors that enhance absorption include:

- **Chew Thoroughly and Eat Mindfully.** Digestion begins in the mouth. Chewing well signals the stomach to release digestive juices and gives enzymes time to begin their work. Eating in a calm, relaxed state activates your parasympathetic "rest and digest" response, improving nutrient uptake.

- **Support Stomach Acid and Enzyme Levels.** Contrary to popular belief, low stomach acid — not high — is often the cause of indigestion. Without adequate acid, proteins can't be properly broken down, and minerals like iron and zinc aren't absorbed efficiently. Bitter herbs, apple cider vinegar, or digestive enzyme supplements can help stimulate this process.

- **Feed Your Microbiome.** Probiotics and fermented foods like sauerkraut, kimchi, kefir, miso soup, and yogurt introduce beneficial bacteria that help metabolize nutrients and strengthen intestinal walls. Pair these with prebiotic fibers (found in onions, garlic, bananas, and asparagus) to feed the good bacteria already living in your gut.

- **Include Healthy Fats.** Vitamins A, D, E, and K are fat-soluble — meaning they require healthy fats for absorption. Add a drizzle of olive oil to vegetables, or enjoy avocado, nuts, and seeds to enhance nutrient uptake naturally.

- **Hydrate Strategically.** Water supports the transport of nutrients through the intestinal lining, but too much water *during* meals can dilute stomach acid. Sip fluids throughout the day, but go easy at mealtime.

- **Repair the Gut Lining.** As previously discussed, nutrients like L-glutamine, zinc carnosine, collagen, and aloe vera help rebuild the intestinal wall and improve its ability to absorb nutrients effectively. This is especially important for anyone recovering from leaky gut, inflammation, or prolonged stress.

Fun Fact: Did you know that when you eat slowly, in gratitude and presence, your body releases more digestive enzymes — up to 40% more according to some studies. The simple act of mindful eating can make your meal more nourishing, even without changing a single ingredient.

Digestive Enzymes: The Unsung Heroes of Gut Health and Absorption. We often talk about the importance of what we eat, but rarely do we consider how well our bodies can *use* what we eat. That process depends heavily on one invisible yet vital force — digestive enzymes. These powerful proteins are the chemical catalysts that break down food into the nutrients our cells need for energy, repair, and renewal. Without enzymes, even the most organic, nutrient-rich meals would pass through us largely unabsorbed. They are the unseen helpers that transform food into fuel, and digestion into nourishment.

Digestive enzymes are produced naturally by the salivary glands, stomach, pancreas, and small intestine. Each one performs a unique task, breaking down a specific nutrient type. Together, they orchestrate a finely tuned process that allows the body to absorb and utilize vitamins, minerals, proteins, fats, and carbohydrates efficiently. However, factors like aging, chronic stress, poor diet, or low stomach acid can reduce enzyme production. When this happens, food isn't fully broken down, leading to bloating, gas, indigestion, fatigue, and nutrient deficiencies, even in those who eat healthfully.

Each digestive enzyme type plays a distinct role in turning food into nourishment. **Amylase** begins the process in the mouth, transforming complex carbohydrates into simple sugars and giving digestion a head start before food even reaches the stomach. **Protease**, sometimes called *peptidase*, works primarily in the stomach and small intestine to break down proteins into amino acids — the building blocks the body uses to repair tissues, create enzymes and hormones, and support the immune system. **Lipase**, secreted by the pancreas, helps digest dietary fats by splitting them into fatty acids and glycerol, which are then absorbed and used for energy and cellular repair.

For those who consume dairy, **lactase** is the enzyme that breaks down lactose, the natural sugar found in milk and cheese; when lactase levels are low, it can lead to bloating or discomfort after dairy consumption. **Cellulase**, though not produced naturally by humans, assists in breaking down the fibrous cell walls of plants and is often included in supplemental blends, especially helpful for those following plant-rich diets. Finally, **maltase** and **sucrase**, produced by the small intestine, complete the digestive process by converting natural sugars such as maltose and sucrose into glucose, the body's most direct source of energy. Together, these enzymes form a sophisticated system that ensures each bite of food can be efficiently transformed into the nourishment and life force your body depends on.

Supplementing with digestive enzymes can be beneficial when experiencing bloating, gas, heaviness after meals, those over 40 (enzyme production naturally declines with age), a history of gallbladder or pancreatic issues, when following a high-protein or high-fat diet, lactose or gluten sensitivities, and when healing from leaky gut or chronic inflammation.

Before reaching for supplements, it helps to encourage your body's own enzyme production:

- **Chew slowly and thoroughly** — saliva releases amylase and signals the stomach to prepare.

- **Eat a mix of raw and cooked foods** — raw fruits and vegetables like pineapple, papaya, mango, kiwi, and sprouts contain living enzymes.

- **Limit water with meals** — too much dilutes stomach acid and weakens enzyme action.

- **Try digestive bitters** — herbs like gentian, dandelion, or artichoke can stimulate stomach acid and pancreatic enzyme release.

- **Relax before eating** — calm breathing before meals activates the parasympathetic "rest and digest" response.

Digestive enzyme supplements are available in plant-based or animal-derived forms. Plant-based enzymes are typically made from papaya, pineapple, or fungal sources and are well-tolerated by most. Animal-derived enzymes (like pancreatin) tend to be stronger and may be used therapeutically. Look for blends that include amylase, protease, lipase, lactase, and cellulase for broad-spectrum support. These are best taken *right before or during meals* to work alongside your body's natural processes. Some formulas also include soothing herbs like ginger, peppermint, or fennel to further ease digestion.

While enzymes are generally safe, it is best to consult a healthcare professional if you have ulcers, gastritis, or reflux (enzymes can irritate the stomach lining), are taking blood thinners (as bromelain and papain may enhance their effects), or have chronic pancreatic conditions or are under medical care.

Heartburn and Indigestion. Because heartburn and indigestion are some of the most common digestive complaints, we will close out with this information. Millions of people experience heartburn or acid reflux every day, and most reach automatically for an antacid to quiet the burn. It's such a common habit that the U.S. antacid market alone generates over $2.5 billion every year, and the global market exceeds $6 billion annually. This simple statistic reveals how many of us are masking digestive symptoms rather than addressing their true cause.

The surprising truth is that most heartburn isn't caused by too much stomach acid. In fact, it's the opposite. When acid levels are *too low* (a condition called hypochlorhydria), food lingers in the stomach longer than it should, leading to fermentation and pressure that pushes acid upward into the esophagus. This creates the burning sensation that feels like "too much acid," but is actually a signal that digestion has slowed down.

Over time, regularly taking antacids or acid-blocking medications can further suppress stomach acid, making digestion even weaker. This can interfere with the absorption of essential nutrients like calcium, magnesium, iron, and vitamin B12, and may contribute to fatigue, brittle bones, and even mood changes. The good news is, there are healthier alternatives for lasting relief. Instead of silencing your body's signals, it's far more effective to support digestion naturally:

- **Stimulate stomach acid** with a teaspoon of apple cider vinegar or a few drops of lemon juice in water before meals.

- **Try digestive bitters** — herbal blends that encourage natural digestive secretions from the stomach and liver.

- **Eat slowly and mindfully**, allowing your body to shift into a calm "rest and digest" state.

- **Avoid lying down immediately after** meals and maintain good posture while eating.

- **Reduce trigger foods** such as processed fats, alcohol, and excess caffeine, which can relax the esophageal sphincter.

When you honor your body's signals and treat the root cause instead of suppressing it, the digestive system gradually regains its natural rhythm. Relief comes not from neutralizing acid, but from restoring balance.

The gut can repair. Give it time and consistency. It's not an overnight process but a gradual return to balance. Most people notice improvement in 4–6 weeks, with deeper changes (like improved skin, mood, and energy) within 3–6 months. Consistency is key; every healing choice you make nourishes your body's ability to rebuild itself from within.

Chapter 7
Food Allergies vs. Food Sensitivities

In today's world, more people than ever are questioning how the foods they eat affect their bodies. Two terms often used interchangeably—*food allergy* and *food sensitivity*—actually describe very different reactions with very different consequences. Knowing the distinction can empower you to identify root causes of discomfort, take back control of your health, and make smarter choices about what you eat.

Food Allergies. A food allergy is an immune system overreaction to a specific food protein. For example, when someone with a peanut allergy eats peanuts, even in tiny amounts, the immune system mistakes the protein as dangerous and releases chemicals like histamine. This can cause immediate, sometimes life-threatening symptoms.

Common symptoms of food allergies:

- Hives, itching, or swelling of the lips/tongue/throat
- Difficulty breathing or wheezing
- Gastrointestinal distress (vomiting, diarrhea, cramping)
- Anaphylaxis (a severe reaction requiring emergency care)

Onset: Symptoms of food allergies usually occur within minutes to two hours after eating the offending food.

Duration: For most people, food allergies are lifelong, especially peanut, tree nut, shellfish, and fish allergies. Some children may outgrow allergies to milk, eggs, wheat, or soy.

Food Sensitivities. Food sensitivities, on the other hand (sometimes called food intolerances) are not immune system mediated. Instead, they involve the digestive system or metabolic processes. Sensitivities may be caused by enzyme deficiencies (such as lactase deficiency in lactose intolerance), difficulty breaking down food compounds (like gluten or histamine), or heightened reactions to chemicals in foods (like caffeine).

Common symptoms of food sensitivities include bloating, gas, cramping, headaches or migraines, brain fog or fatigue, joint pain or skin issues, mood changes

Onset: Unlike allergies, sensitivities can take hours to several days to show up, making them harder to pinpoint.

Duration: Sensitivities are often not permanent. They can be reduced or eliminated by improving gut health, repairing the intestinal lining, balancing the microbiome, or avoiding triggers for a period of time until tolerance improves.

Clearing Allergies vs. Sensitivities

Allergies: At present, the only reliable "treatment" for food allergies is strict avoidance. Emerging therapies like oral immunotherapy (gradually increasing exposure under medical supervision) or NAET may help some people, but allergies generally persist.

NAET (Nambudripad's Allergy Elimination Techniques) is a gentle, non-invasive holistic therapy developed by Dr. Devi Nambudripad in the 1980s to help identify and desensitize the body to allergens and sensitivities. It combines principles from acupuncture, kinesiology (muscle testing), chiropractic adjustments, and nutritional therapy to address the energetic imbalances believed to cause allergic responses.

The purpose of NAET is to retrain the body's nervous system and energy pathways to respond neutrally (rather than reactively) to specific substances. In this method, the practitioner uses muscle testing to detect energetic weaknesses when a person is exposed to a potential allergen (such as a food, chemical, or environmental factor). Gentle stimulation of specific acupuncture or acupressure points is then used to restore balance while the body is exposed to that substance.

Over time and with repeated sessions, NAET aims to help the body reestablish energetic harmony, allowing clients to tolerate previously problematic foods or environmental triggers without symptoms. Many practitioners find it particularly helpful for individuals with multiple sensitivities, digestive issues, chronic fatigue, or immune-related imbalances, as it focuses on the root energetic cause rather than simply managing symptoms.

Sensitivities: These can often be cleared or reduced. Strategies include:

- **Elimination diets** to identify triggers

- **Gut healing protocols** (supporting the microbiome with probiotics, prebiotics, bone broth, and anti-inflammatory foods)

- **Gradual reintroduction** of foods after a period of avoidance

- **Lifestyle support** (stress reduction, adequate sleep, hydration), since these factors impact digestion and sensitivity

The Role of a Food Journal. Because sensitivities often have delayed effects, keeping a detailed food journal is one of the most effective tools for identifying patterns.

Record everything you eat and drink, including portion size, time, and preparation method.

Track symptoms—note timing, intensity, and type (e.g., headache, bloating, rash, fatigue).

Look for patterns—symptoms occurring within 24–72 hours of eating certain foods may indicate sensitivity.

Use elimination diets wisely—remove suspected foods for 2–4 weeks, then reintroduce them one at a time while monitoring symptoms.

Putting It into Practice

If you suspect a food allergy, seek medical testing and supervision. Allergies can be serious and should not be self-tested through reintroduction.

If you suspect a sensitivity, a structured elimination diet and food journal can reveal your unique triggers. Over time, as you repair your gut and rebalance your body, you may find that foods once problematic can be enjoyed again in moderation.

To recap, **f**ood allergies are immediate, immune-driven, and usually lifelong. Food sensitivities are delayed, digestive/metabolic in origin, and often reversible. Keeping a food journal and trying an elimination diet can help you uncover hidden triggers. Gut health plays a major role in whether sensitivities persist or can be healed.

Food Elimination and Reintroduction. To uncover hidden food sensitivities, begin by eliminating common trigger foods such as gluten, dairy, soy, corn, eggs, and processed sugars for 14 to 21 days. During this time, use the *Food Elimination Tracking Form* to record what you eat and note any changes in digestion, energy, mood, or skin. Once symptoms improve or stabilize, slowly reintroduce one food at a time—every three days—while tracking your body's reactions using the *Food Reintroduction Tracking Form*. Pay attention to both immediate and delayed responses, as sensitivities can appear up to 72 hours later. You can download and save these fillable tracking forms by visiting www.ModernWellnessPublishing.com and clicking on the "Table of Contents" tab.

If symptoms return, mark the food as a possible sensitivity and remove the food again for two weeks before adding it back in again. If symptoms reoccur, remove the food from your diet. You may have an allergy as opposed to a sensitivity that doesn't seem to be clearing.

Chapter 8
The Truth About Supplements

In a perfect world, we would get everything our bodies need from fresh, whole foods, sun-ripened produce grown in rich soil, clean water, and unpolluted air. But the modern world is far from perfect. Soils have lost minerals, our food travels long distances, and stress, pollution, and medications all deplete our nutrient reserves. Even those who eat clean and live consciously often fall short in key nutrients, not because of neglect, but because our environment and lifestyles simply demand more than food alone can provide.

This is where supplements come in—not as a replacement for real food, but as allies that help bridge the gap between what we eat and what our cells truly need to thrive. Used wisely, they can replenish what's missing, support the body's repair processes, and provide that extra boost of vitality we need to function at our best.

The Need for Extra Support. No matter how balanced our meals are, it's difficult to rely solely on diet for complete nourishment today. The very soil that grows our food has become depleted of magnesium, zinc, and other vital trace minerals due to industrial farming. Fruits and vegetables lose additional nutrients during storage and transport. Even cooking methods can strip away delicate vitamins. Meanwhile, our bodies are working harder than ever, managing chronic stress, exposure to environmental toxins, and the constant noise of modern life. All of this burns through nutrients faster than we can replace them.

Digestive health also plays a huge role. If the gut is inflamed or the microbiome imbalanced, absorption decreases dramatically. So even the healthiest meal or supplement can go to waste if the body isn't in an optimal state to receive it. Understanding how to choose the right supplements—and in the right form—is essential to making them work for you.

Natural vs. Synthetic: What the Body Recognizes. Not all supplements are created equal. The main difference lies between synthetic and natural, or "whole-food-based," forms. Synthetic vitamins are made in laboratories to imitate natural molecules, but the body doesn't always recognize them in the same way it would nutrients from food. They lack the accompanying enzymes, co-factors, and plant compounds that help the body absorb and utilize them properly. For instance, synthetic ascorbic acid is technically vitamin C, but it's missing the natural bioflavonoids and synergistic compounds found in citrus fruits or acerola cherries that enhance its absorption and effectiveness.

Natural supplements, on the other hand, are derived from plants, herbs, or concentrated food sources. Because they exist in the same matrix nature designed, they tend to be gentler on the system and far more bioavailable, meaning your body can actually absorb and use them. For example, magnesium in its glycinate or citrate form is typically much better tolerated and absorbed than magnesium oxide, which often passes straight through the system unused. In short, the closer a supplement is to its natural form, the better your body understands what to do with it.

The Importance of Absorption. The process of absorption refers to how nutrients move from your digestive tract into your bloodstream, the factor that determines how well your body benefits from what you consume. Factors like gut health, stomach acid levels, and even the timing of when you take your supplements can all make a difference. Fat-soluble vitamins like A, D, E, and K, for instance, absorb best when taken with a meal containing healthy fats. Choosing the right delivery format can make absorption even more effective—and this is where modern science has expanded the possibilities far beyond standard capsules.

The Power of Tinctures. Herbal tinctures are among the oldest and most effective supplement forms known to humankind. Made by steeping herbs in alcohol, glycerin, or vinegar, they extract the plant's active compounds into a concentrated liquid. Because tinctures are absorbed directly under the tongue, they bypass the digestive system entirely, delivering their benefits straight into the bloodstream within minutes.

This makes tinctures ideal for those with compromised digestion, low stomach acid, or difficulty swallowing pills. They're also easily customizable. Herbalists often blend tinctures to support specific needs such as immunity, hormone balance, or sleep. A few drops under the tongue, held briefly before swallowing, can be surprisingly potent. High-quality tinctures are made from organic or wildcrafted herbs and stored away from sunlight to maintain their potency and energetic vitality.

Nano-Sized Supplements: Nutrition at the Cellular Level. In recent years, supplement technology has evolved dramatically. One of the most exciting advancements is the development of nano-sized nutrients, where vitamins, minerals, or herbal compounds are broken down into incredibly small particles—measured in nanometers, or billionths of a meter. These microscopic forms can penetrate cell membranes and enter the bloodstream with remarkable efficiency.

Nano supplements often come in the form of sprays, liquids, or "liposomal" formulas that use tiny fat-like bubbles to protect the nutrients as they travel through the digestive system. The result is faster absorption and greater potency with smaller doses. For example, nano-liposomal vitamin C, glutathione, or curcumin is known for delivering exceptional antioxidant support because it can reach the cells directly instead of being partially lost during digestion.

The key, however, is quality. Not all nano supplements are created equal, and poorly manufactured ones can be unstable or ineffective. Look for brands that use clean, verified nano-delivery methods and transparent ingredient sourcing.

Understanding Ionized Minerals. Another modern approach is ionized supplementation, where minerals are electrically charged into ions, the natural form your body uses to conduct energy. Ionized minerals dissolve instantly in water and enter the bloodstream without needing to be digested. You can think of them as "pre-digested nutrients" that your cells can use immediately.

This is the same principle behind ionized water or electrolyte drinks that restore hydration and electrical balance. When you drink ionic magnesium, calcium, or trace minerals, they help regulate pH, nerve function, and cellular communication. Because the body already operates as an electrical system, these charged particles harmonize beautifully with its natural flow.

Homeopathy: The Subtle Energy of Healing. While most supplements work through biochemical pathways, homeopathy operates on a more subtle, energetic level. Originating from the work of Dr. Samuel Hahnemann in the 1700s, homeopathy is based on the principle of *"like cures* *like"*—the idea that a substance which causes certain symptoms in large doses can, when highly diluted, help the body correct those same symptoms.

Homeopathic remedies are made through repeated dilution and energetic imprinting, a process believed to leave behind a vibrational signature that communicates directly with the body's innate healing intelligence. Rather than adding nutrients, homeopathy reminds the body how to restore its own balance. It's gentle, non-toxic, and safe for all ages, making it an elegant complement to nutritional and energetic wellness practices alike. I have had clients tell me they had success using homeopathy when nothing else worked. There is literally a pellet for nearly every ailment known to man! If you would like to learn more about the amazing world of homeopathy, I would like to refer you to a website that lists every type of remedy available along with educational resources https://homeopathicremediesonline.com.

The Integrative Approach to Supplementation. From whole-food capsules to tinctures, nano-minerals, ionized trace elements, and homeopathic drops, supplements today bridge the gap between science and subtle energy. The goal isn't to take more pills, it's to take the *right* ones, in forms your body can truly use.

When chosen with discernment and paired with clean nutrition, proper hydration, restorative sleep, and emotional balance, supplements become more than nutrients—they become intelligent tools that help the body remember how to thrive. In the end, radiant wellness isn't just about what we put in our bodies—it's about how gracefully our bodies can receive, absorb, and harmonize with what nature and science offer.

Is it Necessary to Take Supplements to Enhance Our Health?

While a balanced, whole-food diet should always be our primary source of nutrition, modern lifestyles, soil depletion, and processed foods often make it difficult to meet all of our micronutrient needs through diet alone. In these cases, taking a high-quality multivitamin can serve as a valuable "nutritional insurance policy," helping to fill in the gaps and support optimal health. Look for a food-based or whole-food multivitamin rather than synthetic isolates, as these are more bioavailable and gentler on the body. For those seeking a more natural alternative, spirulina is an excellent choice—often called *nature's multivitamin*—because it provides a full spectrum of vitamins, minerals, amino acids, and antioxidants in their natural form.

Spirulina offers additional benefits that make it a true superfood:

- **Nutrient Density:** Exceptionally rich in vitamins (especially B-complex, A, K, and E), minerals (iron, magnesium, potassium, zinc), and plant protein.

- **Natural Source of Chlorophyll & Phytonutrients:** Contains chlorophyll, carotenoids, and phycocyanin — powerful antioxidants that protect cells and support detoxification.

- **High Bioavailability:** Its nutrients are easily absorbed because it lacks a tough plant cell wall, allowing the body to assimilate them efficiently.

- **Detoxifying & Alkalizing:** Helps cleanse heavy metals and supports a balanced internal pH for greater energy and vitality.

Adding spirulina to your daily regimen can enhance overall well-being, boost energy, and naturally complement your body's nutritional needs in a clean, sustainable way.

Intuitive Testing

It is important to periodically test yourself on your supplementation. What was once good for you, may not always be good for life. Additionally, when deciding on a new supplement, there are many brands with different compounds and fillers that may not be compatible with your body. Often a healer will recommend a certain product for you because they know it's a good product for what you need, without muscle testing you for it. For example, there are numerous types of probiotics and digestive enzymes, and while they may all be excellent formulas, they may not be the excellent for *you*. Here is where self-testing comes into play. You can test to see if the energy of the product is a good fit for your body's energetic blueprint. There is nothing that is more accurate as the information is coming directly from your body and it's so important to do because a supplement (no matter how good it is) may do you more harm than good if it is not biocompatible with your needs.

- **The Sway Test.** Your innate intuition is a huge benefit if you need immediate guidance on whether a particular food or supplement is healthy for you. I have a lot of fun teaching this to my clients of all ages who are unfamiliar with this practice and watching them get excited when they are feeling and experiencing it working. The sway test is a form of muscle testing where your subconscious mind will communicate with you when you ask it a *yes* or *no* question. You can find videos using this technique on YouTube if you are a visual person. Otherwise, here are the steps: Stand with your body tall and upright. You may leave your arms hanging down or cross them over your chest. You first need to know what your *yes* and *no* answer will look like. For many people, they sway/fall forward for yes. Others may sway backwards for their yes although it's not as common. You may simply ask your body, "what is my 'yes'? Your body should immediately either sway forward or backward. You may also say, what is my 'no' to confirm that you will go the opposite direction. Some people may prefer to get their 'yes' or 'no' by using their name (my name is _____) and using the wrong name to get their 'no'. Once you have established which way you sway for your 'yes', then you can hold the food or product in your hand that you would like to test. For instance, while holding a banana in your hand, ask, "Is this banana good for me?" Your body will provide you with the answer.

- **Traditional Muscle Testing**. This test may be easier for some if they are unable to tap into their intuition when working with the sway test. You can do it on your own or have a friend or family member work with you. Simply hold a supplement in your hand, Extend that arm straight out in front of you. With your other hand, press down on the arm that is holding the supplement. If it holds strong, it is a good fit. If your arm becomes weak, when pushing down on it, that is a clear indication that your body is saying "no thank you" to that particular choice.

Chapter 9
Acidic vs. Alkaline Foods

When foods are digested and metabolized, the nature of their pH level is measured by the ash they create. The term pH stands for parts hydrogen, percentage hydrogen, or potential hydrogen. The pH scale has a range from 0 to 14. A pH reading below seven on the scale indicates increased acidity, and above seven indicates increased alkalinity; seven is neutral. pH is a measurement of the amount of hydrogen ions in a solution. The more hydrogen ions in a solution, the more acidic it is. The body is designed to rid itself of acidity caused by excessive hydrogen and has several ways of doing this. However, a primarily acidic diet can cause our bodies to become overloaded. The higher the acidity level in the body, the less oxygen will be available to the cells. Conversely, the higher the level of alkalinity in the body, more oxygen is available. A well-oxygenated body will have better circulation and a higher energy level than a poorly oxygenated one.

When we refer to pH, we are discussing the amount of hydrogen there is in the body's fluids and tissues. The body maintains a tight pH balance, although pH levels are variable throughout the body for several reasons. For example, the bowels and skin are slightly acidic to guard against harmful bacteria. The urine is typically more acidic and the saliva more alkaline.

In a healthy body, the fluid inside each cell and between cells should be slightly alkaline. The average range of a healthy urine pH is 6.7 – 7.5, and for saliva, it is 6.4 –6.8. The blood pH balance is critical to health and must remain slightly alkaline and in the range of 7.365 – 7.45. The body works hard to maintain a blood pH in this range to prevent a health crisis. However, many people are more acidic than alkaline.

The Importance of an Alkaline Body. Over time, acid can accumulate in tissues, creating destructive imbalances in the body's systems. What's happening is that the cells are being poisoned, causing them to die from oxygen deprivation. Unhealthy cells, such as cancer cells, bacteria, viruses, and other harmful microorganisms, don't survive well in an oxygen-rich environment. In an oxygen-deprived and acidic body, chronic degenerative disease will eventually become evident. Some of the first signs of acid build-up in the body are illnesses such as colds and flus, pain, inflammation, allergies, rashes, and bowel problems such as constipation or diarrhea. An acidic body pH heavy burdens the digestive system, liver, and kidneys and significantly compromises overall health and well-being. According to Traditional Chinese Medicine (TCM), each person generally has a unique weakness in an organ or system that is referred to as our body's constitution. These weakened parts of the body are likely to be the first place where the signs and symptoms of disease will present themselves. In addition, an acidic body is an ideal host for yeasts, molds, fungi, and parasites because these organisms thrive in an oxygen-deprived terrain. Because these organisms are alive, they produce harmful wastes in the body's cells as they derive energy from the body's proteins and fats.

Let's take a look at some common diet choices that will promote a toxic acidic environment.

- <u>Breakfast</u>: Coffee, fried eggs, bacon, bagel with cream cheese.
- <u>Lunch</u>: Roast beef or chicken sandwich on wheat bread with cheese slices, chips or French fries and a soda.
- <u>Dinner</u>: Pizza with pepperoni and sausage with beer and dessert.

As you can see, this type of diet is more common than not. Not a *single* item listed had any alkaline components whatsoever.

Major Causes of Acidity: Toxic chemicals and food additives in processed foods, high amounts of animal protein, dairy, and refined sugar, fried foods, prescription medications, coffee, non-herbal teas, colas, and alcohol, foods containing unhealthy oils, and last but not least, emotional stress.

A body in a chronic state of acidosis sets the stage for chronic, degenerative, and autoimmune health problems. Therefore, the body tries very hard to maintain alkalinity and uses buffering systems that prioritize organ functions and cellular activities to preserve life. We have all heard that toxins are stored in our fat cells. Acidity, being no exception, uses our fat buffering system to prevent acid accumulation in bodily fluids such as the lymph, blood, and between cells (in extracellular fluids). If the body becomes overloaded with acids, it uses fat to bind acids and store them if the acid cannot be eliminated properly. The fat-bound acids may be stored in body parts such as the stomach, thighs, hips, or other areas. The body places the fat-bound acids in these storage areas to protect the vital organs; however, this process promotes obesity.

Tweak the Acidic Meals. Returning to the original scenario, how can we clean up these disastrous meals?

Breakfast: Before breakfast, drink a glass of freshly juiced organic vegetables. If a juicer is not something you have or want, I recommend Organic Suja cold-pressed brand juice only because the sugar content is acceptable. Compare labels to other commercial brands. You may be surprised at the high sugar content. I prefer Suja's Mighty Greens (Apple, celery, cucumber, kale, collard greens, & lemon, ginger, spinach); however, if you want to opt for no added fruit juice, go for the Uber Greens. It tastes better than you might imagine.

Lunch: For lunch, get rid of the soda altogether and have water with lemon. Add sprouts or microgreens, lettuce, tomato and onions to the sandwich.

Dinner: For dinner, add a salad before the pizza. Dress the pizza up with some nutrition in the form of chopped raw garlic, olives, onions and chopped tomato, or sun-dried tomatoes and parsley. Yum!

General Rule of Thumb. Strive for an 80:20 ratio – 80% alkaline foods with 20% acid foods. The most alkaline foods are fresh, raw fruits and vegetables. The goal is not to be perfect but to be aware and to include more of these foods whenever possible.

Start each meal with something raw, such as raw veggie appetizers, vegetable juice or a delicious salad. This not only ensures you get some alkaline foods in your diet but also gives you the digestive enzymes needed to break down any cooked foods that are being served at each meal. If you are traveling and have little choice of what gets served, carry chlorella and spirulina tablets with you, and pop five or six before each meal.

It is a good habit to periodically monitor your progress using acid pH test strips for testing alkaline and acid levels in the body. These test strips can be purchased at Amazon for a reasonable price.

For more information on this topic check out Theodore Baroody's book, *Alkalize or Die: Superior Health Through Proper Alkaline-Acid Balance.*

Chapter 10
The Glycemic Index

The Glycemic Index: Understanding the Hidden Impact of Carbohydrates

Not all carbohydrates are created equal. Some send your blood sugar soaring, while others release energy slowly and steadily, leaving you balanced, satisfied, and energized. The *glycemic index* (GI) is a tool that helps us understand how different foods affect our blood sugar and, ultimately, our health.

The glycemic index measures how quickly a carbohydrate-containing food raises blood glucose after eating. Foods are ranked on a scale from 0 to 100, with pure glucose set at 100. Low GI (0–55) foods cause a gradual rise in blood sugar, medium GI (56–69) create a moderate rise, and high GI (70+) foods cause a sharp spike. This ranking helps us predict the body's response to different foods and guides us in making choices that support steady energy rather than roller-coaster highs and crashes.

Why It Matters

Every time we eat, our blood sugar rises and the pancreas releases insulin, the hormone that helps move glucose into cells for energy. But when we consume too many high-GI foods, insulin levels spike repeatedly. Over time, this pattern can lead to insulin resistance, inflammation, and weight gain. Chronic high blood sugar has been linked to conditions such as type 2 diabetes, cardiovascular disease, hormonal imbalances, accelerated aging due to glycation (sugar binding to proteins and damaging tissues). In short, a diet based on low-glycemic foods helps keep blood sugar stable, protects your metabolism, and supports balanced mood and energy.

The Energy Connection

You've probably felt it — the mid-morning slump after a sugary breakfast or the post-lunch crash that sends you reaching for caffeine. Those dips aren't random. They're the body's reaction to a rapid spike and fall in blood sugar. When glucose drops, so does your energy, focus, and mood. Eating low-GI foods helps sustain vitality by keeping glucose delivery slow and consistent. This is especially important for adrenal and hormonal health, as stable blood sugar reduces the stress response that depletes cortisol and DHEA reserves.

Glycemic Load: The Bigger Picture

While the GI measures *how fast* a food raises blood sugar, *glycemic load (GL)* also considers *how much* carbohydrate it contains. For example, watermelon has a high GI but a low glycemic load because it contains little carbohydrate per serving.
To calculate it:

GL = (GI × grams of carbs per serving) ÷ 100.
Choosing foods with both a low GI and a low GL is ideal for balancing blood sugar and promoting long-term metabolic health.

How to Apply This in Everyday Eating

- **Favor whole foods.** Choose intact grains, beans, lentils, and vegetables over refined carbs.

- **Pair smartly.** Combine carbohydrates with protein, fiber, or healthy fat to slow absorption.

- **Watch portion size.** Even low-GI foods can raise blood sugar if eaten in excess.

- **Be mindful of processing.** The more refined or cooked a food is, the higher its GI tends to be.

- **Choose nature's sweetness.** Fruits like apples, berries, and cherries have a lower GI and come with fiber and antioxidants.

The Mind-Body Connection

Balancing blood sugar is beneficial for both physical and emotional health. Fluctuating glucose levels can cause irritability, anxiety, and brain fog. By stabilizing your internal chemistry, you create a calmer emotional landscape and clearer mental focus. It's another way that what we eat shapes how we feel.

In Essence

The glycemic index empowers us to eat in alignment with our biology — not against it. By choosing foods that release energy gently and nourish us steadily, we cultivate more than metabolic health. We support balance, longevity, and radiant vitality from the inside out.

Category	Low GI (0–55)	Medium GI (56–69)	High GI (70+)
Fruits	Cherries, Apples, Pears, Oranges, Grapefruit, Plums, Berries	Pineapple, Raisins, Mango, Papaya	Watermelon, Dates
Vegetables	Broccoli, Spinach, Kale, Zucchini, Cauliflower, Tomatoes, Carrots (raw)	Sweet Corn, Beets	Potatoes (baked or mashed), Parsnips
Grains & Cereals	Quinoa, Barley, Steel-Cut Oats, Bulgur, Brown Rice, Wild Rice	Couscous, Basmati Rice, Rye Bread	White Bread, Instant Oats, Rice Cakes, Bagels
Legumes	Lentils, Chickpeas, Black Beans, Kidney Beans	Navy Beans, Pinto Beans	None — most legumes are naturally low-GI
Dairy & Alternatives	Milk, Yogurt (unsweetened), Soy Milk, Almond Milk	Low-Fat Fruit Yogurt	Sweetened Yogurt, Ice Cream
Sweeteners	Agave Nectar, Coconut Sugar, Stevia	Honey, Maple Syrup	White Sugar, Corn Syrup, Glucose
Snacks & Processed Foods	Nuts, Seeds, Dark Chocolate (70%+), Popcorn (air-popped)	Granola Bars, Tortilla Chips	Candy, Pastries, White Crackers, Sugary Cereals
Beverages	Green Tea, Herbal Tea, Lemon Water	Fresh Fruit Juice (unsweetened)	Soda, Energy Drinks, Sweetened Beverages

Chapter 11
High Vibrational Foods

The Science of High Vibrational Foods. To maintain good health, we require energy in the form of food, air, and water. Every time we eat specific foods, we absorb the food's energy into our bodies. For that reason, we should focus on eating more high-vibrational foods.

In the late 1930s, André Simoneton, an expert in electromagnetism, was the first to measure the vibration of food based on its electromagnetic field. He researched to define what energetic vibrations benefit or harm the human body. Because the body emits a measurable amount of radiation, his first step in researching the energy of food was to determine the energy of the human body. Radiation from the human body, food, plants, animals, etc., can be shown through color and sound. A healthy body measures between 6200-7200 angstroms. Simoneton determined that to have good health, the human body needs to maintain about 6500 angstroms. When the human body is influenced by lower frequencies emitted by food, it can bring down the vibrational energy of a healthy person, possibly creating disease of the entire body (physically, energetically, spiritually, and emotionally).

The Need for a Nutrient-Dense Diet. We have previously covered several toxic types of edible items posing as foods that should be limited and preferably eliminated. For many people, this will seem undoable and unreasonable if their diet is accustomed to what is referred to as the Standard American Diet (SAD). Which leaves those with the big question, what's left to eat, and what is the importance of eating these nutrient-dense high vibrational foods?

The sad truth is that most of us (including myself) grew up eating anything and everything. We learned to love the taste of sugary foods and candy bars. We grew up eating packaged foods, Captain Crunch and Lucky Charms (because they were so magically delicious), Ho Hos and Ding

Dongs, and clogging our pores with chicken nuggets and fried chicken from the Colonel. Even as adults, we celebrate with cake, cola, ice cream, and alcoholic beverages. There comes a time in our personal evolution when we begin to yearn for true nourishment, when our intuition guides us toward foods that sustain, rather than deplete, our energy. Guided by intuition and an awakening of consciousness, we naturally move toward cleaner, more vibrant foods. And even for those already walking this path, there's always room for small, mindful shifts that bring our diets and our bodies into even greater harmony.

The concept of high-vibrational foods is rooted in holistic medicine and spirituality. While it is nearly impossible for most people to eat a raw vegan diet their entire lives, this type of diet is the winner when it comes to clean eating and high vibrational foods. However, the goal is to incorporate these foods into our diets as much as possible for a healthy balance. According to Simoneton and his findings, he states that the highest vibrations are between 6,500 and 10,000 angstroms, which includes fresh, raw, and juiced vegetables, fruits and vegetables cooked below 70 degrees, cold-pressed oils like olive, coconut, and almond, and essential oils from plants. Also, some foods are higher in energy only if consumed during production, like milk, butter, and eggs, in other words, before pasteurization.

Ideally, food should be used as nourishment and not for pleasure, although eating out at a fine restaurant a couple of times a week is perfectly fine if choosing the best menu items for your health goals. I am an advocate of the diet concept of *fatter days* and *fun days* (within reason) to lighten up the strict confines of the diet throughout the week. Although some of my colleagues would strongly disagree with that philosophy, I believe it is healthier for the body to experience different foods and not constantly eat the same things over and over. Also, getting out to have some fun is always a good thing.

Depending on our diet, food has the power to both heal and make us ill. As Hippocrates, the late Greek physician and philosopher, so eloquently stated, "Let food be thy medicine and medicine be thy food." In fact, the reason why destination healing resorts and centers have a high success rate in reversing cancer and other debilitating diseases is mainly due to the healing diets served to the visiting patients.

The purpose of eating high-quality, nourishing foods is to live in a happy, healthy, lean, light, vibrant body. Disease creates disharmony in the body and causes us to lose our life source energy. Eating foods that are nutritionally dead will break down the body, create disease, pain, depression, brain fog, lack of motivation, illnesses, and a plethora of imbalances within the body. A body in this state lives in a state of confusion and distraction. When we feel bad, we just exist. We don't have the desire to thrive, ascend to our higher states of consciousness, and live a purpose-driven life. The goal is not to live forever but to live as healthily as possible through all stages of life.

High Vibrational Foods Feed the Soul. Now let's get into soul food (and I'm not referring to the delectable fried foods of the south). Simply speaking, high vibrational nutrition is consuming the foods that will nourish our body, mind, and soul with the healing power of nutrient-dense food. High vibrational food is not only essential for the nourishment of our physical bodies but also has a deeper connection to our mental and spiritual well-being by enjoying the peace, joy, and wellness that comes with vibrating at a higher frequency. Just as our bodies require nutrition to function optimally, our souls crave spiritual food for growth and enlightenment. Our bodies function as the temple that encases our soul to experience this lifetime.

High vibrational foods are raw, fresh, whole foods that come directly from the earth and have gathered the sun's energy. They provide mystical life force energy, commonly referred to as Prana, to our bodies. From yogic teachings, Prana comes into the body from the food we eat, the air we breathe, and from absorbing the energies of the earth. Prana aids in formulating the energy of our consciousness, thoughts, and emotions as well as our bodily functions like our breath, digestion, blood flow, and cellular growth and healing. According to the teachings of Paramhansa Yogananda, *"food should be viewed in terms of life force and energy for our sustenance and well-being. Therefore, our diet should include only foods that are easily converted into energy. Our thoughts, actions, and health are generally gauged by the foods we eat, so we need to choose foods that are rich in life force and calming to our nervous system, which help to uplift and expand our consciousness. Foods that are refined, processed and preserved should be avoided because they have lost their life force."*

By choosing to eat foods that have high vibrational energy, we, in turn, are raising our vibration to align with the innate energy of our planet. This aids in strengthening our intuition and our connection to Source energy.

In contrast, low vibrational foods can actually lower our vibration. These types of foods include anything dead, especially factory-farmed meat, fast foods, processed foods, white flour, refined sugar, and genetically modified foods. They provide very little nutrition and very little life force.

Highly processed junk foods drain our energy and lower our vibration, leaving us with low moods or depression, brain fog, sickness, and fatigue. In contrast, high vibrational foods will allow us to feel enlightened, high-spirited, lighter, happier and more focused, full of energy, and fill our bodies with a nutritional powerhouse that is crucial for our wellbeing. The human body is a complete, holistic system operating in harmony with the energy system of the universe. We exchange energy with the rest of the universe all the time. The healthier we are on all levels, the higher our frequency will be.

How Long Do the Good Vibes Last? In other words, how long will the energy last in food, and how much is left in it by the time it gets into our mouth? According to a study conducted by the Leopold Center for Sustainable Agriculture, the average fruit and vegetable travels approximately 1,500 miles, with many being imported from other countries. When food travels such great distances, it loses its vitality & vibration. Fruits and vegetables are at their highest vibration when harvested directly from the plant, tree, or ground and not altered or processed in any way, such as eating a raspberry fresh off the vine or picking kale from your garden. In addition, the longer the distance the food travels, the more energy it can absorb. How the food is treated along its journey also impacts the vibration. Many people handle food during the trip to our table. People have an impact on the energy and vibration of food. If disgruntled people handle the food, it can absorb that energy, further reducing the vibration and vitality of the food. In a nutshell, as soon as fruits and vegetables are picked, they begin to lose their energy charge, and over time, they begin to rot and die. Although most people do not have the land or luxury to grow their own produce, the best fresh produce buying choices are prioritized here: 1) Growing your own produce; 2) Shop at farmers' markets; 3) Shop at co-ops; 4) Local farm-fresh delivery services; 5) Shop at health food stores; 6) Purchase organic produce at commercial grocery stores; and 7) Purchase organic, freshly frozen fruits and produce.

High Vibrational Food Ideas

- **Breakfast Ideas:** Green smoothie (see Chapter 8, #1 Recipe for

Health), acai bowl, steel cut oatmeal with a hint of honey or maple syrup and coconut milk, huevos rancheros with black beans, avocado, salsa, and cilantro, organic plain yogurt (with live probiotics) with blueberries, diced apples baked with cinnamon and coconut sugar

- **Lunch Ideas:** A large salad with chickpeas, cherry tomatoes, avocado with homemade dressing, veggie burger with microgreens, veggie sandwich with alfalfa sprouts, lettuce wraps, seaweed salad

- **Dinner Ideas:** Stir-Fries and Stews (include a variety of vegetables, legumes and spices like turmeric and ginger), homemade soup with a small salad, homemade pizza with fresh toppings and gluten-free crust, vegetable risotto, wild-caught salmon with asparagus, quinoa with mushrooms and steamed or mashed cauliflower, tacos in organic, sprouted, non-GMO corn shells

- **Snacks:** Gogi berries, raw vegetables with hummus or avocado dip, edamame, celery sticks with almond butter, raw nuts, fresh berries, sliced apples with Ceylon cinnamon

Items to Accompany Meals

Spices and herbs: Turmeric, basil, sage, parsley, oregano, cumin, ginger, etc.

Grains: Quinoa, brown rice, wild rice, millet

Seeds and nuts: chia seeds, hemp seeds, sunflower seeds, chopped walnuts, almonds, etc.

Sprouts and microgreens – these are true nutritional powerhouses that provides numerous health benefits and can help boost the immune system.

Fermented foods (good for gut health), seaweed: nori sheets, dried seaweed snacks, dulse flakes, miso soup

High Vibration Food Summary. The highest category contains foods from earth elements consisting of sunlight, pure spring water, fresh air, phytoplankton, chlorella, and spirulina; The second category contains food with high life force energy such as raw chocolate, lemons and limes, goji berries, seaweed, wheatgrass, raw almonds, and herbs; The next category consists of foods from the trees with high life force such as raw nuts, bananas, apples, blueberries, strawberries, raspberries, mangos, grapes, peaches, cherries, pears, oranges, pineapples, coconuts, avocados, and dates. And lastly, foods from the earth. Good examples are kale, spinach, cabbage, carrots, potatoes, sweet potatoes, broccoli, cauliflower, beets, turnips, beans. Cooking will destroy some of the life force.

Chapter 12
Transitioning to a Healthy Diet

"Slow and Steady Wins the Race." -Aesop's Fables-The Tortoise and the Hare

When I first started working as a nutritionist, one of my first clients who wanted to lose about fifty pounds, was all in and immediately started eating her new healthy whole foods diet. She called after a couple of days to tell me that she had to go to the emergency room with intestinal issues. It broke my heart when she told me she was more comfortable going back to her toxic diet.

Whenever transitioning to any type of diet, it is important to transition slowly. In the case of my client, and any other person who regularly eats at McDonald's along with other processed and intestinal clogging foods daily, our bodies become excessively toxic and acidic. Our organs of elimination aren't functioning optimally. Our gut microbiome becomes unbalanced and cannot break down foods properly. When a person makes a radical shift to a clean, whole foods diet of mostly raw fruits and vegetables, it causes our bodies to detoxify. This is a great thing but depending on the amount of pollution and toxic wastes going on in the body, we must do it slowly and steadily.

Cutting out the toxic foods listed in Chapter 3 is the first place to start. If you are not used to eating raw foods, lightly steaming vegetables is a safer bet for your digestive system before transitioning to raw foods. Raw foods can cause gas because they contain high levels of fiber and certain carbohydrates that can be difficult for the body to digest. This, in turn, leads to fermentation in the gut which causes painful gas and bloating. Helping our gut heal from its toxic past with the following supplements will greatly assist in a successful transition to a clean diet.

Binder Supplementation. Slowly detoxing the body to aid the cleansing process of healthy elimination is necessary. When detoxification occurs, it is imperative to incorporate a binder supplement. Since many toxins are fat-soluble, they enter the bile through the intestines, and out of the body through the stool. However, when too many toxins are exiting at once, organs of elimination can't keep up. Our gut lining comprises delicate tissues with veins and nerves that can pick up these toxins and recirculate them. Fortunately for us, a binder supplement has magnetic compounds that will attach to the toxic metals, chemicals, biotoxins, and other impurities that need to exit our bodies, and safely carry them out of the digestive tract without the risk of reabsorption and recirculation. Binders also reduce stress on other elimination and detox organs and help prevent the die-off reaction or healing crisis (also known as a Herxheimer reaction) and uncomfortable detox symptoms.

Probiotics. Probiotics can also be a great asset for improving digestive function by assisting the gut with any imbalance or a deficit of beneficial microbes in the microbiome. When probiotics are consumed either by supplementation or from eating specially prepared fermented foods, they populate the gut with live microorganisms known as good or healthy bacteria. As adults, our guts have around 400 different types of friendly bacteria, which sound like a lot. However, when our diet is not optimal, unfriendly bacteria can take over, causing a condition known as dysbiosis. The goal for healthy gut flora is 80% friendly bacteria and 20% unfriendly bacteria. Taking a probiotic daily will naturally increase the number of beneficial microorganisms in the gut, leaving less space along the intestinal lining for harmful pathogens to attach and multiply.

Digestive Enzymes. Digestive enzymes are extremely helpful in breaking down and digesting food. As we get older, our body makes fewer digestive enzymes. It's not uncommon for people as young as 30 years old to begin to experience digestive issues. Any amount of poorly digested food ferments and putrefies in the digestive tract, which in turn promotes the growth of unfriendly bacteria. When this happens, the toxic waste gets absorbed into the bloodstream, which causes systemic health complications. I suggest a full-spectrum enzyme that will break down each of the food types: Protease (protein), Amylase (starches), Lipase (fats), and Cellulase (sugars).

Please note: Before changing or starting any new diet, it is advised to first consult with your health care specialist for recommendations unique to you and your medical conditions, including testing for food sensitivities.

Chapter 13
#1 Recipe for Health
Smoothies!

One smoothie each morning can be a nutritional powerhouse for your health goals if prepared correctly with a combination of greens, veggies, fruits, proteins, and fats. What better way to start the day than by getting your fruit, vegetables, protein, and healthy fats all in one serving? Expect glowing skin, weight loss, increased energy, detoxification, and vibrant health. In fact, the added nutritional value may help reverse severe medical conditions. However, not all smoothies are created equal. For example, many smoothies offered at restaurants and commercial smoothie bars are packed with fruit juice, sweetened yogurt, sherbet, fruit purees, and sweeteners. When you add all of this up, you have more of a toxic sugar bomb with very little nutritional value posing as a health-promoting smoothie. As an example, if you were to go to the website for Jamba Juice and clicked the Tango Oasis smoothie and searched for its nutritional information, you will learn that it contains 74 grams of sugar! That is the equivalent of eating almost four Snickers candy bars at once. If you make them yourself, you will have control over the ingredients.

You may have heard the term, "breakfast is the most important meal of the day," which may be true if you include a green smoothie in your morning routine. It is the perfect meal to break your fast as it is blended, making it light on the body and the digestive system. The best part is (for fussy eaters), one will never taste the greens and veggies. In fact, I make fun names for all my smoothies, such as tropical delight, strawberry banana, chocolate raspberry truffle, banana blueberry bliss, etc. I recommend smoothies Monday through Friday, allowing variations of different healthy foods to be incorporated over the weekend.

If you are just getting started, it takes a little practice and trial and error until you are ecstatic with the taste and consistency of your smoothies, but it is so worth it. For long-time smoothie drinkers, make it fun and creative so you don't get burned out on them. Discover new ingredients to add to make it even more beneficial to your health. One full-sized blender makes approximately four 16-ounce drinks. Purchase mason jars if you want to store a few days' worth.

PUTTING IT ALL TOGETHER

Choose items from each category below. Those who practice food combining will need to adjust accordingly.

Greens and Veggies: (unlimited to all you can fit.)

Kale, chard, spinach (high in oxalates. Do not use if you are susceptible to kidney stones), mixed bag of super greens, cabbage, Brussels sprouts, broccoli, cauliflower, dandelion greens. Additional throw-ins may include carrot, parsley, celery (best to use with a Vitamix or other commercial blender), cilantro, radishes, etc. Sky's the limit. Be creative!

Protein (choose 1-2)

When using protein powder, ensure it is high quality and organic. Popular protein types are pea, whey, bone broth, hemp, egg whites, and mushroom. Add-ons can include collagen peptides, colostrum, organic plain Greek yogurt, etc.

Fruits – Organic Fresh or Frozen (choose 1-3)

Raspberries, strawberries, blueberries, acai, blackberries, pineapple, ½ banana, apple wedges. Berries are the best choice as they are high in fiber and low in sugar, with raspberries coming in the highest with approximately 9 grams of fiber per serving. I like using frozen fruit as it eliminates the need for ice cubes. Use whole fruit as opposed to fruit juice to get the fiber content.

Healthy Fats (choose 1-2)

Chia seeds (one tsp per serving), MCT oil/powder, flax seeds, avocado, flax seed oil, coconut oil, almond butter, organic raw nuts (almonds, pine nuts, walnuts, macadamia nuts, pumpkin seeds).

Miscellaneous Add-ins: (Optional)

Bee Pollen - Bee pollen has been called nature's most balanced food, and is a storehouse of naturally occurring vitamins, minerals, proteins, amino acids, hormones, and enzymes. Assuming this is not an allergen for you, add one teaspoon per blender serving. Always purchase from the refrigerated section at your health food store.

Super Greens Powders – What better way to add even more benefits to an already perfect meal than by throwing in another teaspoon of antioxidants to the mix. Do your homework and search for a super greens powder online or in a health food store to discover the nutritional benefits. Many contain probiotics and algae, namely chlorella and spirulina.

Chlorella & Spirulina – these popular algae supplements contain numerous nutrients and benefits. In addition, their high protein content contains all essential amino acids that are easily absorbed by the body.

Organic Camu Camu Powder – an excellent source of vitamin C and antioxidant.

Liquid Base: Pure, filtered, or spring water, unsweetened almond milk, coconut water, plain or vanilla coconut milk (unsweetened).

Combining the Contents: Getting started should be fun and a tiny bit overwhelming. However, you will be a pro in no time. Here are a couple of guidelines to help. Fill the bottom of an empty blender with a couple of inches of pure, filtered, or spring water. Add the chia seeds, nuts, bee pollen, other powdered additions, and protein powder. Then add the greens, vegetables, and additional fats. The blender should be ¾ full at this point. Lastly, and lightly, add fruit to sweeten it all up and make it delicious. Add coconut milk or other desired liquid, leaving about one inch from the top.

The following smoothie reference chart can be downloaded by visiting www.ModernWellnessPublishing.com and clicking on "Table of Contents."

Smoothies For Life-Long Health

Just one smoothie each morning can add a nutritional powerhouse to your health goals if prepared with a combination of greens, veggies, fruits, proteins and fats. Expect glowing skin, rapid weight loss, increased energy, detoxification and better health. In fact, the added nutritional value has been known help reverse serious medical conditions.

Fruits (choose 1-3)
- ☐ Raspberries
- ☐ Strawberries
- ☐ Blueberries
- ☐ Acai
- ☐ Blackberries
- ☐ Pineapple
- ☐ ½ Banana
- ☐ Apple wedges

Organic berries are the best choice as they are high in fiber and low in sugar.

Other fruits of your choice may be moderately and occasionally added for flavor.

Greens/Vegetables (unlimited)
- ☐ Spinach
- ☐ Kale
- ☐ Chard
- ☐ Super greens
- ☐ Cabbage
- ☐ Brussel Sprouts
- ☐ Broccoli
- ☐ Romaine
- ☐ Powder Greens

(Optional Additions)
Carrot, celery, parsley, cilantro, radishes, beet, sprouts, dandelion greens, etc.

The sky's the limit. Be creative!

Protein Powders (choose 1)
- ☐ Pea
- ☐ Whey
- ☐ Bone broth
- ☐ Hemp
- ☐ Vegetable-based
- ☐ Egg whites
- ☐ Mushroom/Vegan
- ☐ Maca Powder
- ☐ Other: (optional)
- ☐ Collagen Peptides
- ☐ Colostrum

Optional Additions (organic)
- ☐ Cottage cheese
- ☐ Greek Yogurt (Plain)
- ☐ Probiotic powder

Fats (choose 1-2)
- ☐ Chia seed
- ☐ MCT Oil/Powder
- ☐ Flax seed
- ☐ Avocado
- ☐ Flax seed oil
- ☐ Coconut oil
- ☐ Almond butter
- ☐ Pine nuts
- ☐ Macadamia nuts
- ☐ Pumpkin seeds

Mix all ingredients in a blender with pure, filtered or spring water, unsweetened almond milk or coconut milk until smooth and creamy. Enjoy!

To Your Health!

Chapter 14
Dietary Guidelines

There are nearly 200 different types of diet plans on the market that encompass various approaches to eating, from specific food restrictions like veganism to broader lifestyle changes, including diets based on beliefs or medical reasons. I believe there is only one diet that will work for everyone on the planet. That one diet is the one that is sustainable for YOU. Every diet plan is generally based on one of three primary eating groups: veganism, vegetarianism, or carnivorism.

Veganism is arguably the strictest discipline in both eating and living. It excludes all forms of exploitation and cruelty to animals for food, clothing (silk, wool, leather), or any other purpose. It promotes the development and use of animal-free alternatives to benefit animals, humans, and the environment. In dietary terms, it denotes the practice of dispensing with all products derived wholly or partly from animals, such as eggs, honey, dairy, and all their derivatives, such as cheese, ice cream, collagen, etc. In addition, vegans choose not to support animal exploitation in any form and avoid visiting zoos or aquariums or taking part in dog or horse racing.

Vegetarianism is the theory or practice of eating vegetables, fruits, legumes, and nuts. People choose this diet for ethical, puritan, environmental, or nutritional reasons. Vegetarians who use milk products are sometimes referred to as lacto-vegetarians, and vegetarians who eat eggs are called lacto-ovo vegetarians. Those who exclude land-based meats, like vegetarians, but consume fish and shellfish are called pescatarians.

Plant-based foods are typically high in fiber, vitamins, minerals, antioxidants, and phytonutrients, which are all essential nutrients for optimal health. Moreover, studies have shown that vegetarian diets can reduce the risk of chronic diseases like heart disease, diabetes, and certain types of cancer.

There is a myth that vegans and vegetarians suffer from vitamin deficiencies. The truth is that all the necessary nutrients are found in vegetables, fruits, and nuts when consumed in sufficient amounts; the only exception is vitamin B12. To overcome this potential deficiency, which can cause anemia and other disorders, both vegans and vegetarians need to make sure they are adding foods containing vitamin B12 such as plant-based milks, yogurt or non-dairy yogurt, eggs (vegetarians), shiitake mushrooms, tempeh, nutritional yeast, etc. To ensure sufficient intake, supplement with chlorella and spirulina and sublingual B12. I like Vegan12 by Live Conscious.

The Carnivore Diet includes the flesh and other edible parts of animals, such as cows (beef), pigs (pork), deer (venison), lamb, bison, and birds (chicken, turkey, duck, quail, pheasant, etc.), that humans prepare and consume. In the United States and many other countries, the term "meat" mainly refers to the muscle tissue and fat of mammals and birds. But meat may also include other edible tissues, such as organs.

Just the Guidelines Please!

In holistic health, a diet is not a temporary way of eating until a weight or health goal improves. It is not a dangerous fad diet that tricks your body into behaving differently. It is a way of life. A clean, whole food nutrient-dense way of eating is the only one I recommend. There is no such thing as a one-size-fits-all diet. Every person has a different metabolic makeup, medical needs, and different food sensitivities. The good news is that the following guidelines are universal to good health and should be followed daily.

1. Start every morning by drinking a glass of water. Drink water throughout the day. For added benefit, squeeze in some lemon juice. Continue to drink several more glasses throughout the day. (See the Hydrate chapter for more information.)

2. Remove or limit all toxic food items listed in Chapter 3, Removing Toxins in Our Diet.

3. Limit or remove refined sugar from your diet. Occasional healthy substitutes such as raw honey, coconut sugar, and monk fruit may be used.

4. For healthy digestion, eat fruit on an empty stomach or before meals. Refrain from eating fruit-based desserts after meals.

5. When eating out, skip the fried foods. When cooking with oil at home, only use refined avocado oil, refined coconut oil, refined olive oil, butter, lard, or tallow when using high heat or frying, as these oils have a high smoke point. Use the healthy cold-pressed versions for salad dressings or when cooking without heat.

6. Eat a salad, raw veggies, or vegetable juice before meals.

7. Limit animal protein to 2-4 ounces per meal.

8. When eating animal products, make sure they're organic, cage-free (eggs), grass-fed, and hormone-free.

9. Supplement with digestive enzymes, fermented foods, * or a probiotic supplement, and a gentle binder.

10. Eat a diet rich in organic fruits and vegetables.

11. Incorporate a green smoothie into your daily routine.

12. Always purchase organic raw nuts because they are more nutrient-rich than roasted nuts. Also, soaking nuts for 4-8 hours before eating is not mandatory, however, it improves their digestibility and reduces phytic acid (an anti-nutrient that can hinder the absorption of important minerals such as iron, zinc, and calcium). Soaking also neutralizes enzyme inhibitors, which can interfere with digestion. Skip peanuts as they have a naturally high mold content.

---

* Fermented foods such as kimchi, sauerkraut, and kefir, contain beneficial probiotics; however, people with histamine intolerance, SIBO or candida overgrowth may wish to avoid them as they can have adverse reactions.

Chapter 15
Meat. To Eat or Not to Eat?

We will begin this chapter exploring the age-old question of whether eating meat is unethical and if consuming it will lower our vibration enough to affect our physical, emotional, and spiritual wellbeing. Then we will strictly explore the dietary consequences of eating various types of animal protein and why it should be consumed in moderation.

To begin, these are the questions we will need to ponder:

Is it essential to demonstrate the practice of nonviolence in all areas of our lives? Should we pay as much attention to how animals die as how they live? Does karma come into play for supporting the industry? Is hunting for food acceptable as long as it's not for sport? Will the consumption of meat's denseness and low vibrational nature affect our spiritual practice? As consumers who enjoy eating meat, do we just become oblivious and ignorant, or do we choose to ignore industrial farming practices so that we feel better about eating it? Are we being subtly nudged with uneasiness or guilt when eating meat? Or can we accept the animals' fate, and choose the best quality and humanely raised meat possible, and bless the food we eat, knowing we are getting good and proper nutrition from each bite?

In many cultures, as well as for foodies, the culinary world offers many cuts and preparations of all types of meat, which are considered gourmet delicacies. In contrast, the diet of many is dictated by their religions, spiritual traditions, and culture, which may restrict all or some types of meat, based upon rules of slaughter, cruelty, karma, and physical and spiritual health. Some cultures are simply meat eaters based on their geography and socio-economic status, with no regard to any spiritual consequences.

Many people refrain from eating meat for various reasons, including their intuition that something doesn't feel right about it. Some people choose to eat beef but not veal. A growing number of today's vegetarians refrain from eating meat to improve their health, for a cleaner environment and a better world economy rather than for religious or spiritual concerns. I have known quite a few women who were strict vegetarians who incorporated animal protein back into their diets during their pregnancies. Even those whose vegetarianism is inspired by compassion are often driven more by their conscience than by a spiritual principle.

People who are on a spiritual path often eat meat, yet there are those whose spiritual awakening has led them away from it. Then, there are also those who are not very spiritual but believe that eating meat is wrong. Some spiritual awakenings from eating meat are described as spontaneous occurrences without any physical or environmental factors involved.

Let's examine the beliefs held by religions, spiritual practices, and cultures to determine whether they believe eating meat affects our spiritual growth and, if so, why.

Modern-day Christians may eat meat without restriction. Even though many Christians of the Middle Ages were vegetarians, a meat-eating interpretation of the Bible has slowly become the official position of the Christian church. Although it is said that Jesus taught the virtues of veganism, the scriptures speak of him eating lamb and fish. However, the Seventh-day Adventist Church is a branch of Christianity that strongly supports vegetarianism based upon scripture.

Judaism allows the consumption of meat with some restrictions. The Torah permits eating only those land animals that chew their cud and have cloven hooves. The hare, hyrax, camel, and pig are forbidden because they possess only one of the above characteristics. There are further restrictions on types of fish and birds of prey. The animals that are allowed must also be kosher (a Hebrew word that means *fit for consumption*). This primarily covers how the animal is slaughtered and prepared, with a practice of always keeping milk and meat separate. The belief is that just as there are foods that are good for the body and foods that are harmful, there are foods that nourish the Jewish soul and foods that affect it adversely.

Hinduism and its denominations believe that all of God's creatures are worthy of respect and compassion, regardless of whether they are humans or animals. Therefore, Hinduism encourages vegetarianism, avoiding the eating of any animal meat or flesh. However, not all Hindus choose to practice vegetarianism, and they may adhere to the religion's dietary codes in varying degrees of strictness. For example, some Hindus refrain from eating beef and pork, which are strictly prohibited in the Hindu diet code, but eat other meats. Hindu teachings believe that eating meat is not only detrimental to one's spiritual life but also harmful to one's health and the environment. They believe all our actions, including our food choice, have karmic consequences. By involving oneself in the cycle of inflicting injury, pain and death, even indirectly by eating other creatures, one must, in the future, experience in equal measure the suffering caused.

Jainism practices lacto-vegetarianism and stresses the practice of *ahimsa,* or non-violence. Jains believe in abstaining from meat and honey and avoiding harming any living creatures, including insects. The belief is that harming or killing will cause a harmful karmic reaction.

Taoism is a spiritual tradition that has been around for centuries and its teachings have long emphasized the importance of living in harmony with nature. A key part of this philosophy is a vegetarian diet — one that emphasizes organic, whole foods and avoids animal products. This dietary approach can be beneficial to both our physical health and spiritual well-being, as it reflects an ethical commitment to compassionate living. That said, Taoists are not strictly prohibited from eating meat. However, the traditional Taoist diet emphasizes balance and moderation, allowing consumption of only small amounts of meat on occasion.

Islam stresses kindness, mercy, and compassion for animals. Most Muslims who eat meat follow laws called *Halal,* which allow for "clean" animals that are properly slaughtered. Certain animals are not permitted, depending on how they are killed. Pork is also forbidden in Islam.

Buddhists believe that non-violence and a meat-less diet is crucially important in the successful practice of worship and has a strong tradition of vegetarianism. In some Sutras, Buddha stressed that followers should not eat meat or fish. Many Buddhist monks are strict vegetarians.

Ayurveda is an ancient system of medicine that originated in India more than 3,000 years ago and means "knowledge of life." It is believed that vegetarian food (primarily ripe, raw, or lightly-cooked) is the best for spiritual development. It promotes qualities that support one's journey towards higher states of wellness, mental, and spiritual growth. Such qualities are purity, lightness, balance, and life-giving, providing strength, clarity of mind, compassion, alertness, and calmness.

Yogis strive to live in a manner that is the least harmful to themselves and all other beings. Meat consumption is considered violence against animals, and according to ancient Indian tradition, it is best to choose a vegetarian diet. True yogic belief is to refrain from animal flesh, as they believe it keeps the mind at a lower level of consciousness.

The Blue Zone Centenarians. There are five regions of the world (Okinawa, Japan; Icaria, Greece; Sardinia, Italy; Nicoya, Costa Rica; and Loma Linda, California) where people often live to be over 100. They have been tracked and studied to determine why these zones have such happy, healthy people. The common thread was their diet as well as a sense of community. This information has led to books, numerous periodicals, documentaries, and cookbooks. In a nutshell, their diet primarily consists of 90% plant-based foods. They limit animal protein to no more than one small serving per day. Some staples are beans, greens, yams, sweet potatoes, fruits, nuts, and seeds. Those who eat bread choose sourdough or whole wheat. While people in four of the five blue zones consume meat, they do so sparingly, using it as a celebratory food, a small side, or a way to flavor dishes as opposed to the California Blue Zone which consists of the Seventh-day Adventists who refer to their diet as *The Garden of Eden Diet*, which omits animal protein and wine. This is based on Biblical guidance as stated in Genesis 1:29, "I give you every seed-bearing plant on the face of the whole earth and every tree that has fruit with seed in it. They will be yours for food." There is also a strong compassion for kindness to animals. They believe in God's new kingdom, we will go back to this Garden of Eden diet, where there will be peace and no killing of animals.

In conclusion, many controversies, factors, and personal beliefs come into play on the topic of eating animal protein. The question of whether eating meat affects our health has been a topic of debate for centuries, with different spiritual traditions offering varying opinions on the matter. The energy and vibrations present in the food we eat play a significant role in shaping our overall energetic state and consciousness. How could it not? Another concept that affects the energy of our food is our thoughts about it. In your heart and soul, if you are at peace with eating meat, perfect! If you are feeling guilty, shameful, unhealthy, or would like to quit but haven't quite pulled the plug yet, there may be a struggle going on with your inner guidance. If we do not feel good about our diet, this can disrupt everything from our digestive system to our emotional health and will no doubt lower the vibration of every bite because of our thoughts about it.

As a nutritionist, I must present all information so that each person can make their own decision about what feels right for them at each stage of their lives based on their inner guidance, regardless of what others on a spiritual path are doing, or what religious leaders or gurus are telling us to do. I do believe animal protein is dense and causes a certain heaviness. As such, one who doesn't eat much meat may find themselves craving a burger or a steak after an energetic healing session or intense meditation practice to help with grounding (FYI, eating root vegetables will also help with this process). Although, I do believe consuming commercially raised animals can lower our vibrational frequency due to their chemical components. However, when choosing organic grass-fed meats in small quantities, we will be consuming much healthier nutrient-rich protein.

For those who enjoy meals that contain meat, here are some guidelines that are important to follow:

1. Avoid *all* commercial factory-farmed animal products. The conditions are harsh and cruel. It is safe to say that all commercial industrial farmers whose goal is to provide an end-product with the best profits for their shareholders are using growth hormones and antibiotics to make livestock grow faster and survive the crowded, unsanitary conditions of factory farms to keep them plump and disease-free. It is believed that our bodies will also be absorbing what they eat and are injected with, including stress hormones from their conditions. All fast-food establishments are serving these low-quality products, as well as many restaurants, unless otherwise noted on their menus.

2. Know your farmer. I don't necessarily mean to know them personally but know their farming practices. Talk to them at the farmer's markets. Were they humanely treated? Did the farmers care for their animals' health and well-being? Are their cows pasture-raised? Did they roam in a stress-free, peaceful environment? Were they fed high-quality plant-based, non-GMO feeds to ensure their utmost health?

3. Rule of thumb for the best health practices: Meat eaters should consume the highest quality lean meat. Look for the words, organic, grass fed, pasture raised, no added hormones, etc. Limit intake to 2-4 ounces per serving per day.

4. Always bless your meat before eating. Give thanks to the animal for

the nourishment it is providing.

Let's shift over to the dietary aspects of eating animal protein and explore why consuming too much can have several detrimental health effects. And yes, the type of meat matters significantly. Here's a breakdown:

Kidney Strain. High protein intake, especially from animal sources, increases the workload on the kidneys. Over time, this may contribute to kidney damage or accelerate kidney disease in those already at risk.

Bone Health Concerns. Diets very high in animal protein can increase calcium excretion in urine, potentially weakening bones over time if calcium intake isn't adequate.

Heart and Vascular Issues. Many animal proteins, especially red and processed meats, are high in saturated fats and cholesterol, which may raise LDL ("bad") cholesterol and increase the risk of heart disease, stroke, and atherosclerosis.

Cancer Risk. Processed meats (bacon, hot dogs, sausages, deli meats) and red meats have been linked to higher rates of colorectal and stomach cancer, partly due to compounds formed during processing and high-heat cooking (nitrosamines, heterocyclic amines, polycyclic aromatic hydrocarbons).

Inflammation and Aging. Excess methionine (an amino acid abundant in meat) and advanced glycation end-products (AGEs) formed in cooking may promote inflammation, oxidative stress, and accelerate aging.

Digestive Issues. Diets too heavy in animal protein often lack fiber (since fiber only comes from plants), leading to constipation, gut microbiome imbalances, and reduced colon health.

Types of Animal Protein are a Factor

Processed Meats (bacon, sausages, deli meats). Highest risk. Classified by the WHO as *Group 1 carcinogens*. Strongly linked to cancer, cardiovascular disease, and type 2 diabetes.

Red Meat (beef, pork, lamb). Moderately high risk when consumed in excess. Increases heart disease and colorectal cancer risk. The risk worsens if meat is charred or grilled at high temperatures.

White Meat (chicken, turkey). Leaner than red meat and lower in saturated fat. Considered safer in moderation but fried or heavily processed versions still carry risks.

Fish & Seafood. Generally healthier, especially fatty fish like salmon, sardines, and mackerel, which provide omega-3 fatty acids beneficial for heart and brain health. Risks include mercury in large predatory fish (tuna, swordfish) and contamination depending on sourcing.

Dairy & Eggs. Moderation is key. Eggs are nutrient-dense but can raise cholesterol in sensitive individuals. High-fat dairy can contribute to cardiovascular risk, but fermented dairy (yogurt, kefir) may support gut health.

Balance & Recommendations

- Limit processed meats or avoid entirely.
- Keep red meat moderate (occasional, small portions, grass-fed if possible).
- Emphasize plant proteins (beans, lentils, quinoa, nuts, seeds) to balance the diet with fiber, antioxidants, and phytonutrients.
- Choose healthier cooking methods (baking, steaming, slow cooking) over frying, grilling, or charring.
- Pair animal protein with plenty of vegetables and fiber to offset acidity and support digestion.

Chapter 16
Hydration for Vitality

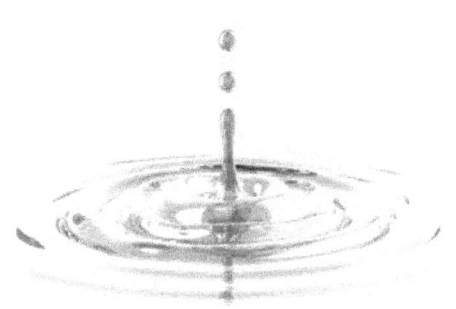

WATER, the Essence of Life...

Water is our most important life source. Water is essential for all functions within our cellular structure. If we don't get enough, we simply cannot survive. Our bodies are composed of almost 75% water. The brain is made of nearly 90% water. With so many choices of beverages available to us, we can often take water for granted, and neglect to drink this vital source our bodies so desperately crave. Dehydration is a serious but silent epidemic. Many ailments we experience can be improved once we increase our water consumption. The chart below displays a handful of risk factors directly related to dehydration if not corrected:

> Constipation · Arthritis · Chronic fatigue · Irritability
> Headaches · Brain fog · Insomnia · Mood swings
> Wrinkles · Heart issues · Weight gain · Bad breath
> Body aches · Poor concentration · Depression · Toxicity
> Organ failure · Chronic illnesses · Death

How Much Water Should We Drink Daily? As a baseline, divide your body weight in half to get your required daily ounces. For example, if your weight is 140 pounds, your baseline water requirement is 70 ounces of water daily (close to nine 8oz glasses of water). In addition to your daily requirements, add an extra glass of water if:

Sweating from being in a sauna, prolonged periods in the sun, fever, exercise or other physical activity; when consuming coffee; when consuming alcohol; if illness or diarrhea is present; and when traveling.

Upon waking and before eating or consuming coffee or tea in the morning, drink a full glass of water without ice. This will help to replace fluids lost overnight, detox your body, and get your hydration off to a good start. Keeping a glass of water on your nightstand is a good practice.

Drink water throughout the day. Never wait until you are thirsty. Your body is already dehydrated if it is thirsty. Yes, it is possible and dangerous to drink too much water. However, don't be overconcerned about this. For most of the population, this will never be an issue.

For those who don't find drinking water particularly enjoyable, try creating your own spa-infused water by adding your choice of lemon or lime slices, orange, strawberries, or cucumber. Be creative!

Water Filtration Systems. Never drink tap water from the faucet. It not only tastes bad, but it is not a good idea for our health or for our pets' health. The Environmental Working Group has found over 140 contaminants in tap water. In addition, over the past decade, studies have shown that pharmaceuticals, like prescription and over-the-counter drugs, are being found in tap water. Some of the most common drugs found in water are antibiotics, anti-depressants, birth control pills, seizure medication, cancer treatments, painkillers, tranquilizers, and cholesterol-lowering compounds. Every home must have some kind of filtration system. While any type of filtering system is better than drinking tap water, some are better than others. Don't get caught up in the hype of claims made by companies selling expensive alkaline filtration systems. I like reverse osmosis with a mineral filter, so the minerals that were removed in the filtration process are added back. Do your research and decide which filtering system is best for you. As an alternative, water stores are a good choice to purchase and fill up 3-gallon or 5-gallon containers of water that sit on a stand. Water delivery is also convenient. Always opt for spring water when it's available.

Bottled Water. Many bottled waters that claim to be *purified* are filtered tap water and not the best quality choice. Be careful when purchasing and consuming bottled water. The preferred choice is spring water, and preferably ones sold in a glass bottle, as plastic toxins may leach from the plastic bottles, especially when exposed to sunlight. Try to get in the habit of filling a water bottle from your water filter before leaving the house.

Water Absorption. Some people can drink an adequate amount of water daily and yet feel dehydrated and dried out. If this is the case, water absorption may be an issue. If you are drinking water, and it is going right through you, and you still feel thirsty or dehydrated, it could be from a mineral imbalance. Adding electrolytes can help with this issue. Electrolytes are minerals that dissolve in water that carry an electric charge.

There are many commercial products, such as sports drinks and powders or packets to add to water that are not the healthiest choices, and some that are good can be quite expensive. Some excellent recommendations to supercharge your water for better absorption and health are as follows:

-e-Lyte by Body Bio – highest electrolyte concentration available formulated with the three ingredients you need to bring electrolytes back to the perfect pH balance - Sodium, Potassium and Magnesium.

-Trace Minerals 40,000 Volts Concentrate Supplement Drops for Electrolyte Support is a top-of-the-line product. Although the package says it's unflavored, it does add a slight taste that may be objectionable to some people. Experiment with various brands until you find one that you enjoy in water.

-Cellfood Liquid Drops boost oxygen, energy, endurance, and hydration. Add eight drops to a glass of water. It has a slight lemony taste.

-Redmond Real Salt contains over 60 natural trace minerals – beneficial to pinch a little in a glass of water or place a dash under your tongue before drinking a glass of water.

-Structured water is a type of energetically enhanced water that is run through a swirling vortex. This process mimics the process of spring water trickling down mountain streams over sand, pebbles, and rocks, collecting minerals as it travels. In other words, the water becomes charged with electrical energy from the Earth's magnetism and cosmic energy. Structured water is more easily absorbed by the body than regular water due to its unique molecular arrangement, which allows for better penetration into cells and improved hydration at the cellular level. There are many types of structured water units on the market. After extensive research, I have found the handheld units available at www.StructuredWaterUnit.com to be a relatively inexpensive and high-quality option.

Enhanced Water. Our bodies require a fair amount of water daily. Since we are already drinking it, why not enhance its healing benefits for superior health and energy from one of the sources below?

-Fulvic Humic Acid drops. These electrically charged drops provide our bodies with polysaccharides and more oxygen for better energy, stronger immunity, and better digestion. Just five drops in a glass of water are nothing short of a medical miracle for our cellular health. Although it turns the water slightly brown, there is no taste. I highly recommend them for daily use.

-Liquid chlorophyll drops are a game changer for energy, antioxidant enhancement, good digestion, and detoxification support.

-pHenomenal Water is a company that takes its water seriously. Instead of adding mineral content to add alkalinity, their unique process literally transforms the water by pulling out the acidity turning it into alkaline water. The drops are tasteless.

-Shilajit drops. Shilajit resin is a sticky substance found primarily in the rocks of the Himalayas. It develops over centuries from the slow decomposition of plants. The anti-aging claims are extensive, from prevention of Alzheimer's, treating chronic fatigue, treating anemia, improving bone density, raising testosterone levels, protecting against free radicals, and much more. It may be worth enduring the funky taste for the benefits.

-Hydrogen water (H2). Water infused with hydrogen gas is said to have phenomenal benefits for anti-aging, preventing over 200 health conditions. It requires the purchase of a hydrogen generator that takes approximately 10 minutes to create an eight-ounce glass of hydrogen water. It must be consumed immediately before the gas dissipates. Generators that produce 5000 ppb are required for the therapeutic effects mentioned. If you don't have the time or discipline required for this daily routine, molecular hydrogen tables can be purchased and added to a glass of water.

Chapter 17
Daily Detox

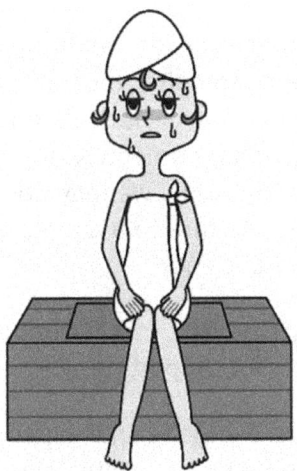

Wouldn't it be ideal if all we needed to do were to eat clean foods, breathe clean air, apply chemical-free toiletries, and not have to concern ourselves with detoxification? Unfortunately, no matter how hard we try, we have had a lifetime of toxic exposure, where chemicals, molds, and heavy metals often don't leave our system. In addition, we will continue to acquire many more daily. Our bodies have an impeccable skill to detox what we eat, drink, breathe, and absorb through our skin. However, an overabundance of chemical exposure can create a backup, and our detoxification pathways cannot keep up unless we step in to help. We will discuss safe, mild, and effective methods to help our bodies cope daily. Before starting any detoxification protocols, it is always best to consult your doctor or health care provider to see if you are a good candidate.

The body's organs of elimination include the liver, kidneys, lungs, skin, lymphatic system, and digestive system, which encompasses the colon. Within each category, there are effective ways to keep our bodies functioning optimally.

Liver: The liver is our primary means of detoxification and is responsible for converting toxins into waste products and cleansing the blood.

- Water. Drinking plenty of pure water throughout the day is one of the healthiest things we can do for our bodies to aid in the detoxification process.

- Castor oil packs. This is an easy do-it-yourself home remedy that involves applying a cloth soaked in castor oil over your liver with a heating pad that aids in detoxifying the body.

- Cilantro. Cilantro is excellent for supporting detoxification by breaking down and promoting the transport of heavy metals from the body through the liver. In fact, cilantro has been coined as the poor man's chelation treatment. As food, it is a healthy addition for flavor, but for detoxing, we may need a stronger dose. I like adding the liquid tincture to a couple of ounces of water, and down it goes. Nice and easy!

- Supplements such as milk thistle, turmeric, and dandelion root are effective herbs for supporting liver health.

Kidneys: The kidneys filter the blood and help remove the toxins through urination. The health of our kidneys is integral to the health of the rest of our body. It's essential for our kidneys to function properly to avoid toxic buildup and formation of stones.

- Hydration. Of course, when it comes to the kidneys, drinking plenty of water is our best source.

- Kidney-cleansing teas. Teas known for detoxing the kidneys are dandelion, moringa, hydrangea, Sambong, cranberry or any combination thereof.

- Calcium-rich foods. Eating sufficient amounts of calcium helps to bind and break down oxalates, the naturally occurring compounds in foods (especially spinach) that contribute to kidney stones if our bodies are unable to break them down.

- Homeopathic remedies for kidney stones. According to the National Kidney Foundation, approximately 1 in 10 people will develop kidney stones in their lifetime. Natural remedies such as Kidney Stone Clear by NativeRemedies will keep this situation at bay. Other remedies for urinary tract health include Chanca Piedra (known as the *stone breaker*) and hydrangea root extract are herbal remedies that claim to be effective.

- D-mannose. Low doses are safe to take daily to prevent bacteria from sticking to the walls of the urinary tract and causing infection – a life-savor for those who get UTIs.

Lungs: The lungs help eliminate toxins and wastes through respiration by removing carbon dioxide and other volatile substances. It would be nice to say go out and breathe in fresh air; however, we don't know where our air has been. We breathe in many particles from wildfires, strong winds that carry fungal spores, pesticides, herbicides, exhaust, and other air pollutants, including particles and metals expelled from the chemical spraying (What goes up, must come down.). Giving our lungs a little love will help to clear out what doesn't belong there and will help prevent respiratory illnesses.

- Mullein Leaf Extract. It's a great detox for the lungs. I like the tincture form. Put 30 drops in a few ounces of water. It's safe to use daily. It is recommended as a preventative, especially for city dwellers, people with airborne allergies, asthma, COPD, or those who feel like they are coming down with a respiratory virus.

- Air filters. Studies show that indoor air can be more polluted than outdoor air. A high-quality air filter can remove particles that would normally go directly into your lungs such as smoke, dust, pollen, mold, viruses and bacteria. Purchasing a model with a charcoal (carbon) filter will also help remove gaseous pollutants such as volatile organic compounds or ozone.

- Steam therapy. Steam inhalers deliver water vapor to the airways to help the lungs drain mucus-containing toxins.

- Neti pot. Neti pots are small teapot-looking devices that use saline for nasal irrigation to remove mucus by washing out allergens, irritants, and debris from the nasal passages.

- Halotherapy (salt therapy). Salt air has impressive health benefits for our lungs and respiratory system. Many spas and wellness centers offer salt caves, salt rooms, and halo generators where you can go in, relax, and breathe in the salt air. Whenever possible, walk along the seashore and breathe in the benefits. For those who can't get to the ocean or the spa, Himalayan salt inhalers can be purchased inexpensively on Amazon.

Skin: Our skin is our largest organ, protecting us from environmental toxins and excreting them through sweating.

- Sweating in an Infrared Sauna. Sweating is my favorite and, in my opinion, the absolute best way to detox heavy metals, plastics, pesticides, mold and mycotoxins, impurities, and toxic chemicals out of the body. As you know, for our protection, our fat cells are a storage reservoir for accumulated toxins. Regular use of the sauna will help to pull these toxins out, which, as a bonus, will provide weight loss and fat reduction. However, the process takes time. Remember to be patient as these toxins may have been stored for decades. It is ideal to have one in the home. There are all sizes, spaces, and price variations for all types of homes and budgets so there should be no excuses when it comes to getting a good, detoxifying sweat. Some options are a single person sauna. Clearlight and Medical Saunas are excellent brands but on the pricy side. If going for lower-priced models, make sure the manufacturer's product claims to be low in EMFs. Other types of infrared devices are sauna domes or portable sauna tents. Therasage makes a great product. An infrared sauna blanket can be purchased from Amazon for under $200. If purchasing one is not a viable option, using a gym's wet/steam sauna is also effective. I recommend 30-minute sessions, depending on how long it takes before the first drop of sweat begins to fall. The average for most people to break a sweat is around 8-12 minutes. I recommend a full 20 minutes of flowing sweat. Because we lose valuable minerals from sweating, it is important to replenish them by adding fulvic acid drops, Cellfood drops, or other forms of electrolytes into your post-session's 16-ounce glass of water. More info on this topic is covered next in the Hydrate chapter.

Lymphatic system: Our lymph system is part of our immune system and is crucial for filtering waste and toxins from the body. Lymphatic fluid is carried through a complex network to lymph nodes where toxins, metabolic waste products, fat, and excess liquid are filtered and purified by regional lymph nodes. In a congested lymphatic system, the fluid is thick, sticky, and laden with toxins that cannot be properly eliminated. Keeping our lymph functioning properly is not so much a detox, but a drainage protocol. Usually with proper hydration and exercise, the average healthy person doesn't require reinforcements, although the following protocols are still a good practice for increasing circulation.

- Rebounding or jumping on a mini trampoline for five minutes a day. Whole body vibration machines fall into this category.

- Dry skin brushing. There are several articles on the internet discussing methods to do this correctly. However, just lightly stroking your skin for a few minutes before showering with a natural bristle brush throughout your body, including the palms and bottoms of your feet, towards your heart, will do the trick.

- An inversion table. Hanging upside down for 3-5 minutes has a number of health benefits to improve back pain, increase flexibility, and enhance circulation. It also aids in detoxification by moving the lymph fluid through the body by using gravity in reverse. Instead of gravity moving lymph fluid to the feet, it moves it away from the feet and toward the upper body. Then, when you are no longer inverted, gravity helps move lymph fluid again. For those who are athletically able, headstands fall into this category.

- Lymph massages. Those who enjoy massages also find them good for stimulating the lymph system. There are massage therapists who have been trained in giving lymph massages. In addition, many wellness clinics offer electronic lymph drainage with a special machine designed to detoxify the body from a buildup of lymph toxins. It is relaxing and feels slightly tingly.

Colon: The colon is the last part of the digestive tract extending from the small intestine to the anus, where waste products and toxins are removed through our stools. The liver and other organs will remain congested as long as the colon remains toxic. The goal is to keep things moving along (and out).

- Coffee enemas. Coffee enemas can cleanse the colon and remove toxins. While I have not done one myself, clients and colleagues rave about them. Check with your doctor to learn if that may be a good solution for you.

- Colonics. Colon hydrotherapy, or colonics, is a method of rinsing the colon with warm water using a tube, a machine and an operator. Fecal build-up, mucus plagues, and harmful bacteria are expelled, allowing essential nutrients to be better absorbed. In addition, I have had clients report the loss of an excess of 10-20 pounds. It is essential to take probiotics after doing colon hydrotherapy to replenish the gut with the good bacteria that was lost in the process. For those who cringe at the thought or refuse colonics, oxy-powder or MagO supplementation can practically accomplish the same thing by utilizing an oxygen-based method to rid the intestinal tract of toxins and waste.

- Intestinal Cleanse Supplements. There are numerous products on the market that will do the trick. One recommendation is Dr. Schulze's Intestinal Formula #1 or #2. These types of colon-cleansing formulas are specifically designed to remove the accumulation of impurities and toxic buildup that we have been collecting and storing in our intestines for years.

- Binders. A binder supplement uses its magnetic action to bind to toxins in the intestines in preparation to be expelled. They are needed so toxins do not recirculate back into the body. Some good ones are as follows: Fruit pectins (apple or citrus) are helpful for binding metals, such as mercury and lead, and also mycotoxins from mold exposure. Activated charcoal mops up biofilm once it has been broken up, preventing the released bacteria, parasites, and other biotoxins from being reabsorbed by the gut lining. Chlorella is also a good, gentle binder that can effectively bind to heavy metals, pesticides, herbicides, molds, mycotoxins, and VOCs. Chlorella also helps to detox exposure from any type of radiation such as X-rays or airport security.

Oral Hygiene: According to the National Library of Medicine, the oral cavity has the second largest and most diverse microbiota after the gut, harboring over 700 species of bacteria and nurturing numerous microorganisms, which include bacteria, fungi, viruses, and protozoa. The mouth, with its various niches, is an exceptionally complex habitat where microbes colonize the hard surfaces of the teeth and the soft tissues of the oral mucosa.

In addition to being the initiation point of digestion, the oral microbiome is crucial in maintaining oral and systemic health. Even though it is not an area of elimination that warrants a detox, we should include it here as it is undoubtedly an area that can use some extra attention aside from simply brushing twice a day. In addition, the condition of our oral health is systemic, which means that it affects not only our teeth and gums but also our overall health.

- Oil Pulling. Oil pulling is a holistic ancient Ayurvedic practice originating in India over 3000 years ago. It involves swishing oil around in your mouth for 10-20 minutes. It is said to promote oral health by pulling out harmful bacteria. According to a study published in PubMed, it also helps to eliminate *streptococcus mutans* levels in the mouth, which is often associated with tooth decay, plaque, and gum disease. In addition, it has the merits of offering a full spectrum of health benefits by detoxifying the body due to the reduction of harmful bacteria-related conditions that can be transferred to the body. It is a simple process. Use 1-2 teaspoons of your choice of sesame oil, coconut oil, or sunflower oil in the morning on an empty stomach. Swish the oil around in the mouth for ten minutes. Spit the used oil into the trash and follow with rinsing and brushing your teeth.

- Electric toothbrushes. Electric toothbrushes are far superior to using manual toothbrushes. Users of manual toothbrushes can only accomplish up to 300 strokes per minute. Oscillating toothbrushes can provide 2,500 to 7,500 strokes per minute, offering a better cleaning to prevent decay and gum disease. They are extremely affordable, starting at only $35.

- Tongue Scrapers. The tongue is part of the mouth and, as such, also contains harmful bacteria, food particles and other debris that brushing (even with an electric toothbrush) cannot do as effectively.

- Oral Probiotic. Oral hygiene probiotic lozenges help inhibit undesirable bacteria in the mouth and support optimal oral health. FLORASSIST by Health Extension is a good and affordable brand.

Up to this point we have discussed ways to detox invaders out of our body. However, detox could also include prevention. In comes the Wein Mini-Mate Wearable Air Purifier. I am including this item for its uniqueness and innovative health benefits. This ultra-light wearable purifier uses closed-field plasma and ionic wind technology to create a personal "clean-air zone" around your breathing space. It is filter-free, silent, and maintenance-free, making it ideal for travel, offices, and tight indoor spaces. The device helps reduce airborne particles (dust, pollen, mold spores, smoke, viruses) down to sizes as small as 0.04 microns. This item is especially useful in crowded or polluted environments and perfect for traveling on airplanes and public transportation. To explore how this technology works, you can visit their website at www.weinproducts.com.

Chapter 18
Exercise Your Way to Radiance

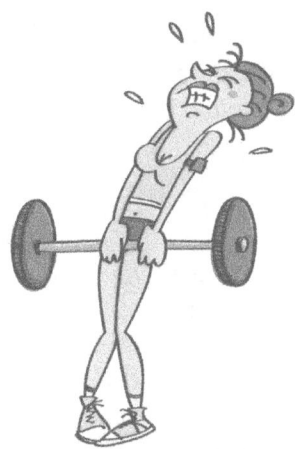

Look ten years younger with regular exercise! Okay, now that I have your attention on a topic many people put off—because they're too busy, think it's boring, or simply feel lazy—let's talk about the wonderful benefits of movement (yes, exercise!).

Without regular exercise and proper nutrition, muscles may become rigid with age and lose tone. Bones become more brittle and may break more easily. Overall height decreases, mainly because the trunk and spine shorten. Breakdown of the joints may lead to inflammation, pain, stiffness, and deformity. In other words, if we don't keep the equipment moving, our muscles will atrophy. Living our best life at every stage of our journey on this planet will be much easier and more rewarding if we are vibrant, happy, healthy, and pain-free. The good news is if we have gotten lazy or lost our zest for exercise, it is never too late to start.

At approximately 30 years of age, bone and muscle mass naturally decline. Bone density decreases and muscle tissue is replaced with fibrous tissue, leading to conditions like sarcopenia and osteoporosis. Sarcopenia is the gradual loss of muscle mass, strength, and function that occurs with aging. It affects our gait, balance, and overall ability to perform daily tasks. Osteoporosis is a skeletal disorder characterized by low bone mass, deterioration of bone tissue leading to more porous bones, and consequent increase in fracture risk. It is the most common reason for broken bones and hip fractures as we get older. In addition to reduced physical activity, both menopause and andropause cause declining levels of hormones like testosterone and insulin-like growth factor (IGF-1) which contribute to muscle loss.

According to the Centers for Disease Control (CDC), all older adults, both men and women, can benefit from regular, moderate physical activity, including those experiencing medical conditions such as arthritis, heart disease, obesity, and high blood pressure.

Key Benefits of Exercise

- Better stamina. By boosting our cardiovascular function, we strengthen our lungs and airways and improve our stamina.

- Mood enhancement. Our bodies release endorphins when we exercise, decreasing the cortisol stress hormone. Endorphins are the body's natural feel-good chemicals, and when released during exercise, they trigger a positive feeling and naturally boost our mood. Aside from endorphins, exercise releases adrenaline, serotonin, and dopamine hormones. These hormones work together to make us feel good and positive. Endorphins, along with serotonin and dopamine, are known as happiness hormones that help ease anxiety and depression.

- Pain relief. Endorphins, also known as the body's painkillers, are released by the brain and nervous system to combat discomfort and pain.

- Bone health. Exercise keeps bones strong by stimulating bone tissue to grow and increase in density, mainly through weight-bearing activities like running, strength training, or lifting weights.

- Muscle growth. Engaging in muscle-strengthening activities is beneficial for building or maintaining muscle mass and strength.

- Better energy. Exercise increases energy levels by improving cardiovascular efficiency, allowing the heart and lungs to deliver oxygen and nutrients more effectively to muscles and tissues. Additionally, regular physical activity enhances mitochondrial function in cells, which keeps us looking younger and feeling vibrant.

- Brain health. Exercise improves brain health and memory by increasing blood flow to the brain, which helps deliver more oxygen and nutrients needed for brain function. It also boosts the production of a brain-derived neurotrophic factor (BDNF) protein. BDNF supports the growth and survival of brain cells, enhances the connections between them, and helps improve memory and learning.

- Weight management. Regular exercise helps burn calories, which is crucial for maintaining or achieving a healthy weight. It also boosts our metabolism, making it easier to manage our weight over time. This also helps to keep blood sugar levels intact to prevent diabetes.

- Improved immune system. Exercise strengthens the immune system and helps regulate key health markers such as blood pressure and cholesterol levels. Regular physical activity lowers the risk of many types of illnesses.

- Connection. Participating in group exercise is excellent for emotional health for all age groups. A sense of community significantly impacts our health and well-being by fostering social connections, reducing stress and isolation, and ultimately leading to better happiness and interest, keeping us motivated to keep showing up to exercise. Having community involvement is the one thing that centenarians (people living 100+ years) all have in common.

How Much Exercise Do We Need?

As a general rule of thumb, set a goal to get at least 30 minutes of exercise daily. Any extra is a bonus. If time constraints are an issue, you can break up the 30-minute workout into more manageable 10-minute blocks and still reap enormous benefits. If a day is missed, shoot for an hour of exercise the following day. Setting realistic goals to avoid burnout will provide long-term success. Discovering what you enjoy doing will also keep the interest, whether it's dancing to your favorite tunes, working out with a friend, or enjoying the serenity of exercising outdoors. Keep it interesting by doing different types of exercise throughout the week.

Types of Exercise

Stretching. Stretching is an absolute must before exercise; however, incorporating a morning stretching routine upon waking improves flexibility, reduces stiffness, increases blood flow, and boosts energy and mood. 10-15 minutes will do the trick. However, this does not count toward our 30-minute daily goal.

Brisk walking or light jogging. Brisk walking is considered moderate-intensity exercise at a pace of 3-4 miles per hour. It is an excellent choice for exercise as it provides all the health benefits of exercise and is low impact on the joints. It can be done wherever you are whether on a treadmill or out on a nature walk, in city streets, or along the seashore.

Rebounding. According to a NASA study, jumping on a trampoline has been said to produce the benefits of 30 minutes of regular exercise in only 10 minutes. It is excellent for strengthening the cardiovascular system as well as detoxing the lymphatic drainage system. Jumping rope is also great exercise, although a bit more strenuous. It's like rebounding on steroids.

Strength training. Strength training can be done with resistance bands, light or heavy weights, and gym equipment. This choice is *imperative* for the stimulating bone health and building and maintaining strong muscles, improving metabolism, and improving body composition.

Yoga and Pilates. Both yoga and Pilates are considered mind-body fitness modalities and are exceptionally good for improved flexibility, enhanced core strength, and balance. These mindfulness practices help to incorporate controlled movements and breathing techniques.

Tai chi and Qigong Both tai chi and Qigong are gentle forms of exercise that combine slow, flowing movements with deep breathing and meditation. Their wide range of physical and mental health benefits make them perfect for all ages and fitness levels. Give them both a try to see which one best suits your enjoyment.

Dancing. Dancing may be your preferred choice of exercise if you get bored easily. It combines cardio with strength training and toning. With all the choices from Zumba, hip-hop, ballroom, barre, step aerobics, salsa, belly dancing, jazzercise, jazz, tap, flamenco, and line dancing, you will have a lot of fun exploring the ones you like the best. For something a little different, you may want to try ecstatic dance, a free-form practice focusing on self-expression and connection to achieve a meditative state, and to experiencing a sense of ecstasy.

Team sports. Any number of sports, such as softball leagues, pickleball, tennis, volleyball, and the like, will be sure to get you moving while having fun at the same time.

Swimming. Swimming is a favorite for many people because of its low impact. Moving to the resistance of the water is excellent for cardiovascular health, while working out nearly every muscle in your body.

Hiking. This one is so enjoyable it's hard to believe it counts as exercise. The uneven terrain keeps everything engaged. Walking uphill engages the glutes, quads, hamstrings, and calves, while going downhill gets the ankles, hips, and core. In addition, connecting with nature improves our mental health and well-being.

Biking. Cycling is a favorite for its low impact on the joints. Whether we exercise on a stationary bike, a mountain bike, cruiser, or a road bike (sorry, electric bikes don't count), all the health benefits are there including the improvement of stamina and endurance. It's also good for body toning as well.

Stair Climbing and Hills. Wherever there are multiple public stairs, you will more than likely find people flocking to them to work out. It's an excellent way to get outdoors while reaping the enormous benefits of interval training.

Floor Exercises. Whether you're stuck in a hotel room without a gym or have time constraints, incorporating a few sets of push-ups into any daily activity has tremendous benefits for upper body strength, targeting the chest, shoulders, triceps, and biceps. Squats and lunges will target the other half by working out the quads, hamstrings, and glutes. Throw a few sit-ups or crunches to strengthen the core, and you've got it made.

Pep Talk: Keep Moving Forward

Movement is life and your body was designed to move. Every step, every stretch, every conscious breath awakens the energy within you and reminds your cells that you are alive and thriving. You don't have to run marathons or spend hours in the gym; what matters most is consistency and joy in motion. Dance, walk, swim, stretch, flow — whatever moves your spirit moves your body, too.

When you make movement a daily ritual, you're not just building strength and flexibility, you're signaling to your body that you choose vitality, longevity, and freedom. So, keep moving, keep glowing, and remember: the energy you invest in your body today becomes the radiance you carry into tomorrow.

Chapter 19
Sleep Yourself Well

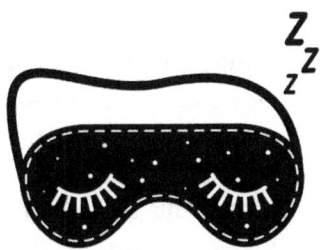

Recent studies show that one in three people worldwide struggles with poor-quality sleep. Our body's natural production of GABA and melatonin declines as we age. Combined with our rapidly aging society and technological innovations designed to maximize our screen time, it is no wonder we're a bit sleep deprived.

Regularly getting a good night's sleep is one of the best gifts you can give your body in terms of physical and mental health. Although we spend one-third of our lives sleeping, this is one of the areas in our lives that often gets taken for granted. The biological science of sleep is quite fascinating. Let's go back to our school days for a refresher course when we first learned all about what happens after we lie our heads on our pillows and turn out the lights.

The Four Stages of Sleep

Each night, our bodies experience four stages of sleep, known as our sleep architecture. The first stage is referred to as N1. This is where we start drifting off to sleep. This stage is a very light sleep that we can easily be awakened from. During N1, our brain waves start to slow down, creating a pattern of theta waves. This phase can last between one and five minutes before moving on to the next phase.

N2 is considered a light sleep stage where the body starts to relax. The brain activity slows down while still showing brief bursts of activity called sleep spindles or short bursts of rhythmic brain activity. It is the stage where most of our sleep time is spent, making up around half of our total sleep duration. Our heart rate, breathing, and body temperature continue to decrease. It is harder for us to wake up from this stage than the N1 stage. This stage is crucial for transitioning into deeper sleep stages, and it is essential for memory consolidation. This stage can last anywhere from 10 minutes to one hour.

The N3 deep sleep stage is considered the most restorative sleep stage. It is critical for restoring our body and mind. This is where delta wave activity processes our memories and experiences from the day while our body releases growth hormones to repair muscle tissue, regrow bone cells, and strengthen the immune system. This stage is the most difficult to wake up in. Older adults tend to experience less N3 sleep compared to younger people. This stage lasts between 20 to 40 minutes.

REM (rapid eye movement) is the final sleep stage, characterized by rapid eye movements behind closed eyelids. During this stage, the brain is almost as active as it is when it's awake. Evidence shows that REM sleep contributes to insightful thinking, creativity, memory, and vivid dreams. It also stimulates the areas of the brain that help with learning and memory, brain repair, processing emotional experiences, and transferring short-term memories into long-term memories. The first REM period of the night lasts about 10 minutes, and each subsequent period gets longer. The final REM period can last up to an hour.

These four stages repeat in 90–110-minute increments throughout the night. Depending on how long we sleep, the body may go through this cycle four to six times each evening. The ideal amount of time to sleep for ages 18 and older is 7-8 hours.

Napping. Napping can be healthy when it's done correctly. Short naps, approximately 20-30 minutes, can improve alertness, cognitive function, and overall performance, especially when experiencing temporary sleeplessness. However, longer or frequent naps can disrupt nighttime sleep, so set your timers.

The Importance of Getting Enough Sleep. Anyone who has been deprived of a night's sleep or has had severe insomnia knows how difficult it is to function the next day. However, when it happens regularly, we begin to run into problems. Not getting enough sleep drains your mental abilities and puts your physical health at risk. Science has linked inadequate sleep with a number of health problems, including weight gain, chronic stress, poor aging, and a weakened immune system.

Recommendations for a Good Night's Sleep

- Avoid television, cell phones, iPads, and computers one hour before sleep. If this can't be avoided, apply a blue-blocking screen on your laptop and cell phone, or wear blue-blocking glasses. Reading a good old-fashioned paperback book is a good practice for creating relaxation and sleepiness (no thriller novels, of course!).
- Eat at least 2-3 hours before going to sleep.
- Sleep in a dark room or no more than a nightlight with yellow, orange, or red wavelengths.
- Put your cell phone on airplane mode or turn it off. Make sure your head is away from any electrical outlets.
- You should have a routine where you go to bed around the same time each night and get up at the same time every morning.
- Don't sleep with an electric blanket. They emit EMFs and also affect your sleep rhythm as it disrupts your body's natural temperature, causing lighter sleep and more awakenings.
- Use an air filter if windows are closed while sleeping.
- Keep the room at a temperature of around 65 degrees.
- Cut out all caffeinated beverages eight hours before your regular bedtime.

Insomnia. According to the Sleep Foundation, a person with healthy sleep patterns typically takes 10-20 minutes to fall asleep and ideally stay asleep until morning. Any type of variation to this pattern is considered a form of insomnia. Short-term insomnia is a brief episode of difficulty sleeping due to a stressful life event. Chronic insomnia is a long-term pattern of having trouble falling asleep or staying asleep at least three nights per week for three months or longer. Most of us can fit into at least one of the categories of insomnia from time to time.

- Sleep onset insomnia describes difficulty falling asleep at the beginning of the night. Most people with sleep onset problems aren't able to fall asleep even after spending 20-30 minutes in bed. The inability to fall asleep means that a person with insomnia of this nature has reduced total sleep time and can feel the effects of that lack of sleep the next day.

- Sleep maintenance insomnia describes an inability to stay asleep through the night. Most often, this means waking up at least once during the night and struggling to get back to sleep for at least 20-30 minutes. The fragmented sleep associated with poor sleep maintenance means a decrease in sleep quantity and creates a higher chance of daytime sleepiness or sluggishness.

- Terminal insomnia, also called late insomnia, occurs when we wake up too early and aren't able to get back to sleep. Early morning awakening insomnia typically involves waking an hour or more before we would normally get up. This pattern can impair our physical and mental function the next day.

- Mixed insomnia applies to those who have a combination of problems related to sleep-onset, sleep maintenance, and early morning awakenings.

- Comorbid insomnia or secondary insomnia arises as a result of another condition such as stress, anxiety, depression, sleep apnea, or digestion issues.

Sleep Aids and Tricks. Natural sleep aids can help promote deep, restful sleep without feeling groggy the next morning. However, what works for some people may not work for others. A little trial and error will go a long way to find an effective solution.

Binaural Beats: Binaural beats played through a headset program the brain to relax. It works by influencing brain wave activity through entrainment, where the brain naturally synchronizes with the frequency of the beat, essentially tuning itself to a slower, more relaxed state when exposed to a chosen frequency. Studies suggest that listening to binaural beats at specific frequencies, like delta waves, may help improve sleep quality by increasing deep sleep duration and reducing sleep latency (time to fall asleep). Hemi-Sync tracks get good reviews. You can explore different titles from their website and listen to samples before purchasing tracks. They are inexpensive and can be directly downloaded to your iPhone or iPad. Binaural beats for sleep can also be found on YouTube for free (search term: binaural beats for sleep), or the Pandora, or Amazon Music apps.

Words: If you are having trouble falling asleep, lie on your back. Place one hand on your stomach and the other on your heart. Take three slow deep breaths and begin thinking of positive words (calm, relaxed, peaceful, love, grateful, etc...) until you doze off. Repeating positive words or affirmations before sleep influences our gene expression through epigenetic mechanisms allowing our mental state to change from overactive to relaxed, thereby having a measurable effect on our body's sleep patterns.

A Relaxing Bath: If you enjoy baths, a nice warm bath using Epsom salts and lavender essential oil has a calming scent, that helps the brain produce neurotransmitters that reduce stress and promote sleep. Soaking your feet in warm water with Epsom salts is also relaxing and beneficial before bedtime.

Breathwork: Deep breathing directly affects the nervous system and promotes relaxation, reduces stress, and increases melatonin production. There are various breathwork techniques, however, Box Breathing is one that is simple and instantly helps calm the nervous system and promotes relaxation for falling asleep quickly. Box Breathing is also called Square Breathing because of the four different steps involved and each step being carried out for the duration of four counts (seconds). It is also called 4-4-4-4 Breathing, Four Square Breathing, or Equal Breathing. By simply laying on your back, take four slow breaths in through your nostrils, hold it in for four seconds, then slowly exhale through your mouth for four seconds, and then wait four seconds before the next round of breathing.

The Military Sleep Method can help you fall asleep quickly. By focusing on each of your muscle groups, starting with your forehead, down to your eyes, nose, cheeks, mouth, and jaw. Focus on one part at a time, breathing deeply and letting go of any muscle tension you're holding there. Relax your tongue and the muscles around your eyes. Proceed to your shoulders, arms, and fingers; work your way down your chest, abdomen, and pelvis. Then, focus on one leg, relaxing your thigh, knee, calf, ankle, foot, and toes. Do the same with your other leg. If you're still awake at this point, close it out by clearing your mind. Try to visualize a calming scene, such as a cork bobbing up and down in a body of water.

Calm.com is a subscription-based app that offers bedtime stories (yes, for adults!), sleep meditations, music and soundscapes that promote a restful night's sleep.

Herbs and Such: Experimentation is the key. What works for some may not work for others.

- Chamomile is a flowering plant that has been used for centuries for its medicinal properties. It is beneficial for anxiety and sleep. Chamomile contains apigenin, an antioxidant that may bind to receptors in the brain to promote relaxation, reduce anxiety, and improve sleep quality. While it is most common as a tea, a liquid tincture is available and can be added in 2 ounces of water before bed.

- Melatonin, which is naturally produced by the pineal gland, can also be taken as a supplement. Crossing through the blood-brain barrier, a small dose 30 minutes to 1 hour before bedtime can help promote sleepiness, allowing for a healthy sleep pattern. Dosage is critical with melatonin. No more than 3 mg is advisable for sleep regularity, as larger doses often cause grogginess.

- L-tryptophan is the compound in turkey that is well known for its sedative effects. This amino acid is utilized to produce melatonin along with calming neurotransmitters which help quiet any anxious thoughts keeping you awake. In this way, L-tryptophan helps improve the quality and reliability of our sleep cycles.

- Passion flower (passiflora incarnata) is an herbal remedy used for its calming and sedative properties. It contains several organic compounds that promote relaxation by increasing the body's natural production of GABA. When taken at night before bed, it may help people fall asleep faster and increase their time spent in the deeper, more restorative stages of slow-wave sleep.

- Magnolia bark contains two organic compounds, magnolol and honokiol, which help activate the GABA receptors in the brain. Through this mechanism, magnolia bark enhances the calming effects of our natural GABA production and keeps our minds at peace throughout the night, improving sleep quality and limiting interruptions.

- L-Theanine is an amino acid that occurs naturally in tea leaves. It has been found to reduce anxiety and promote the level of relaxation in the brain needed for high quality restful sleep.

- Lemon balm, often used in sleep-inducing tea blends, contains natural compounds that help quiet your mind by inhibiting an enzyme that normally breaks down and recycles GABA. In this way, this member of the mint family helps maintain higher levels of GABA longer, allowing your mind to remain peaceful and relaxed for a full night of deep, restful sleep.

- Drink concoctions: Sleepytime tea blends and Calm Magnesium may be helpful in promoting a restful night's sleep.

- Homeopathic remedies. I have had clients tell me that homeopathic remedies worked for them for various issues when nothing else did. There are numerous variations out there that pinpoint special sleep needs. I highly recommend exploring this avenue especially if none of the others listed have worked for you (search: homeopathic remedies for sleep).

Chapter 20
Holistic Dental Health & Biological Dentistry

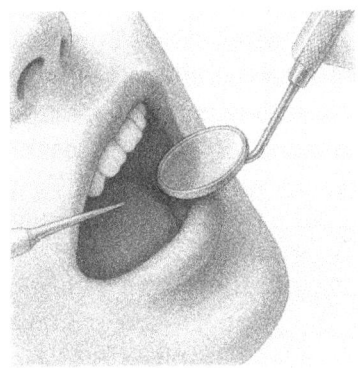

We often think of our teeth as isolated structures for chewing and smiling. Yet in holistic medicine, the mouth is viewed as a powerful mirror of the body's internal health. Each tooth is connected to an energetic pathway known as a meridian — the same meridian system mapped out in Traditional Chinese Medicine. Through these channels, every tooth corresponds to a specific organ, gland, and even emotional pattern.

For instance, the upper front teeth are linked to the kidneys and bladder; the canines correspond to the liver and gallbladder; the premolars and molars are connected with the lungs, stomach, and intestines. This means that an infection, root canal, or even chronic inflammation in one tooth can energetically influence the health of the organ along that same pathway. Conversely, if an organ system becomes weakened or congested, you may begin to experience sensitivity, decay, or pain in its corresponding tooth, even if your dental X-rays appear normal.

The Silent Energy of Infected Teeth. When a tooth dies, whether from trauma or deep decay, the tissue inside begins to decompose. Root canal therapy attempts to save that tooth by removing the infected pulp and sealing the canal. However, no matter how skillfully performed, a root-canaled tooth is no longer alive. Without its blood and lymph flow, it can harbor residual bacteria and energetic stagnation. Studies have shown that microscopic pathogens can linger in the tiny dentinal tubules, creating chronic low-grade infections that may not show up in routine tests but can quietly burden the immune system.

Biological and holistic dentists refer to this as an "energetic blockage." The body constantly fights to wall off the toxic influence, diverting immune resources and contributing to fatigue, inflammation, and even distant organ dysfunction. For example, people with recurrent sinus issues sometimes discover that a previously root-canaled upper molar sits directly on the meridian line for the sinuses. Others with chronic digestive problems have found the source tied to a long-forgotten abscess on a tooth connected to the stomach meridian.

A Tale of Two Dental Philosophies. Conventional dentistry, grounded in mechanical repair, often views the tooth strictly in terms of structure and infection control. From this perspective, if a root canal looks clean on an X-ray, the problem is considered resolved. Biological dentistry, however, integrates energetic, microbial, and systemic perspectives. Practitioners may use thermography, muscle testing, or electro-dermal screening to assess subtle imbalances. They focus not only on the tooth itself, but on how the mouth interacts with the rest of the body's electrical and lymphatic systems.

Mainstream dentistry typically does not endorse the tooth–organ connection model, as it's not widely supported by conventional research methodologies. Yet many patients have experienced profound health improvements after addressing chronic dental infections, removing metal amalgams, or extracting root-canaled teeth that tested as energetically "dead." These case observations have driven a growing field of integrative dental medicine — a bridge between science and energy healing.

Bringing the Mouth Back into Balance. Holistic dental care blends modern hygiene with energetic awareness. Oil pulling, ozone therapy, infrared light, and herbal mouth rinses can all support oral detoxification. Working with a biological dentist can help identify hidden infections, metal sensitivities, or jaw cavitations that may be affecting your energy flow and organ function. When you approach dental health as part of your whole-body wellness plan, you reclaim one of the most powerful — and overlooked — keys to lifelong vitality.

The Root Cause Documentary. Back in 2018, I started to get an influx of new clients hiring me to run their bioenergetic scans. All of them seemed to have an unusual interest in their tooth results. Finally, around the fifth client who seemed anxious to learn how their teeth checked out, I finally asked, "What's going on? Why does everyone suddenly have so much interest in their teeth?" I learned they had just watched a documentary called *The Root Cause*.

This film delves into the theory that chronic infections from root canals can contribute to a wide range of systemic health issues — from fatigue and autoimmune conditions to heart disease and even cancer. It interviews biological dentists, holistic doctors, and patients who experienced major health turnarounds after addressing infected or root-canaled teeth.

While the film sparked enormous curiosity and opened new conversations about dental toxicity, it also drew sharp criticism from the conventional dental community, who dismissed many of its claims as unproven or alarmist. Major streaming platforms temporarily removed the film following pressure from dental organizations.

Regardless of one's stance, *The Root Cause* highlights an important point: there is still much we don't fully understand about the mouth's influence on whole-body health. It invites viewers to consider the possibility that dental health is not an isolated system, but part of a larger energetic and biological network. For readers exploring holistic wellness, it serves as a reminder to stay curious, research broadly, and make decisions based on both science and intuition.

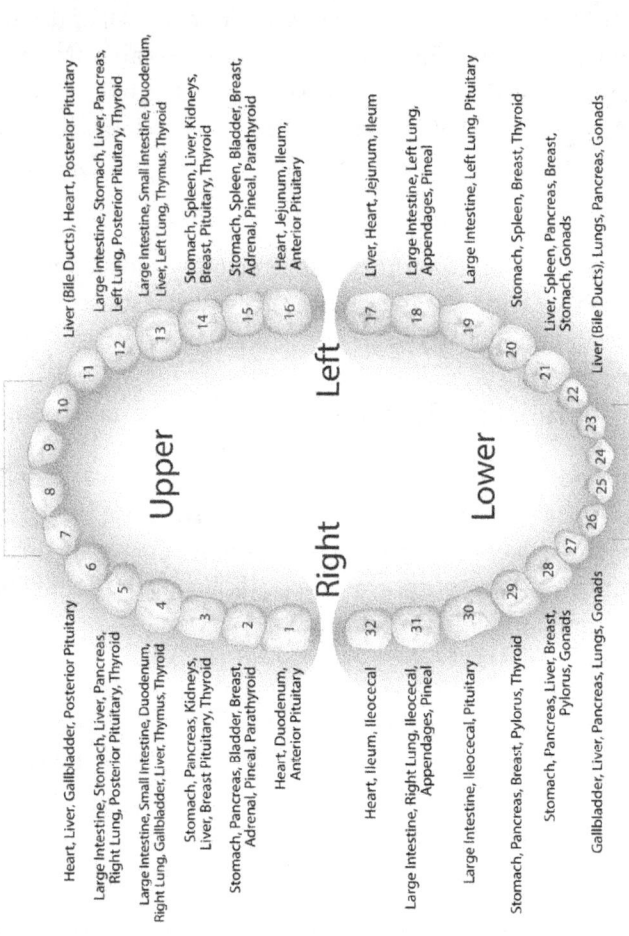

PART TWO: THE MIND-BODY CONNECTION

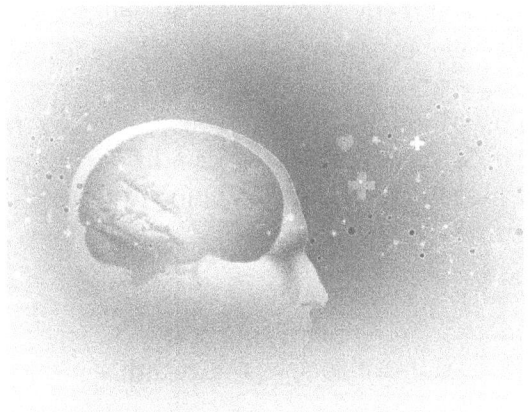

In the radiant wellness journey, our inner world is everything because what we think, feel, and believe is intimately woven into our health, our happiness, and the life we are co-creating.

Science now shows that the mind-body link is real and powerful: thoughts, emotions, and beliefs don't just live in your head—they spark chemical, neurological, and physical responses throughout your whole being. When your mind is aligned, your body flourishes; when it isn't, discomfort, illness, and low-vibration patterns can take root.

In this section we'll explore how both positive and negative thoughts and feelings can shape everything from immune strength to stress levels as well as our happiness and joy. Emotional states like hope, calm and optimism are shown to boost well-being, while chronic stress, worry and fear put measurable strain on the body systems.

We will also be guided into self-reflection, the gentle, honest exploration of our own inner emotional landscape. This practice reveals which emotional beliefs or patterns no longer serve, allowing us to release what's weighing us down, and make space for what supports our vitality.

All of this fits within the holistic lifestyle: body, mind and spirit are not separate but intimately connected. By nurturing that integration, through awareness, emotional clarity and intentional choice, radiant wellbeing becomes not a distant goal, but your everyday lived reality.

The Roots of Mind-Body Health

The idea of mind–body health suggesting that thoughts, emotions, and spiritual awareness directly affect physical well-being, has become a well-accepted part of mainstream wellness and medicine. Its roots reach back thousands of years and travel through many cultures, philosophies, and scientific breakthroughs. To understand how we arrived at today's integrative and holistic approaches, we can trace a lineage from ancient practices to 19th-century metaphysical pioneers, early psychosomatic medicine researchers, as well as modern science that brought these concepts into existence.

Long before modern science, civilizations across the globe recognized that mental and spiritual states shape physical health.

- **Ayurveda in India** taught that balance of body, mind, and spirit maintains health and that disease arises when this harmony is lost.

- **Traditional Chinese Medicine** emphasized the flow of *qi* and the influence of emotions on the organs, using acupuncture, herbs, and meditation.

- **Greek and Roman thinkers** like Hippocrates and Galen highlighted the healing power of nature and the role of temperament and lifestyle.

- **Indigenous and shamanic traditions** worldwide integrated ritual, prayer, and energy work to treat illness as a disturbance of the soul.

These traditions laid a philosophical groundwork that would resurface centuries later in new forms.

The metaphysical surge in the 1800s saw an explosion of interest in health's mental and spiritual dimensions, giving birth to what became known as the New Thought movement.

- **Phineas Parkhurst Quimby** (1802-1866), often called the father of New Thought, proposed that illness originates in erroneous beliefs. By correcting thought patterns and aligning with divine truth, he taught, the body could heal.

- **Emma Curtis Hopkins** (1849-1925) trained many influential teachers and helped spread the belief that the mind creates health.

- **Ralph Waldo Emerson** and **Wallace Wattles** wove philosophy and positive thinking into an empowering message: the inner life determines outer reality.

At the dawn of the 20th century, attention turned to the scientific study of how thoughts influence the body.

- **Émile Coué** (1857-1926) pioneered *autosuggestion*, the idea that repeating positive phrases "Every day, in every way, I'm getting better and better" could trigger real physical improvement.

- **Sigmund Freud** (1856-1939) and early psychoanalysts explored how unconscious conflict manifests as physical symptoms, giving rise to the concept of psychosomatic medicine.

- **Carl Jung** (1875-1961) illuminated the link between psyche and body, teaching that true healing arises from integrating the conscious and unconscious self as a journey toward inner harmony and wholeness.

- **Wilhelm Reich** (1897-1957): A student of Freud, Reich linked chronic muscular tension ("body armor") to suppressed emotions, suggesting this could eventually cause illness.

These thinkers laid the groundwork for a truly integrative understanding of health, blending psychology with the realities of the body.

The spiritual teachers of the early 20th century also brought wisdom from Eastern traditions to Western audiences.

- **Paramahansa Yogananda** (1893–1952), through *Autobiography of a Yogi*, introduced yoga, meditation, and the unity of body, mind, and soul to millions.
- **Edgar Cayce** (1877–1945), the "sleeping prophet," provided intuitive readings that combined diet, prayer, and energy balancing.
- **Pierre Teilhard de Chardin** (1881–1955), a French Jesuit priest, scientist, and philosopher, envisioned human evolution as a spiritual unfolding that connected matter and spirit.

These figures reinforced the ancient insight that spiritual consciousness and physical vitality are inseparable.

Louise Hay (1926–2017) stepped into this innovative ground, and her book *You Can Heal Your Life* (1984) became a cultural phenomenon. As a motivational speaker and author, she offered millions an accessible path of affirmations, self-love, and forgiveness. She suggested that unresolved emotions and negative self-talk could contribute to illness and that consciously choosing loving thoughts could catalyze healing. Her work drew directly from New Thought and autosuggestion traditions, but her plain spoken style and focus on emotional self-healing made these ideas resonate with a broad audience.

By the mid-20th century, science joined the conversation, and scientific research began to validate what spiritual traditions had long taught.

- **George Engel's biopsychosocial model** reframed disease as the interaction of biological, psychological, and social factors in health.
- **Herbert Benson, M.D.**, is considered to be the modern medical pioneer who brought mind-body health to mainstream Western healthcare. At Harvard, his research demonstrated that meditation and simple breathing practices trigger the "relaxation response," reducing blood pressure and stress. In 1975, he published a book of the same name.
- **Jon Kabat-Zinn** built on this with Mindfulness-Based Stress Reduction (MBSR), making meditation a mainstream therapeutic tool.

- **Dr. Candace Pert:** Neuroscientist and author of *Molecules of Emotion*, demonstrated that neuropeptides (emotion-related molecules) interact with the immune and endocrine systems—providing biological evidence for the emotion–illness link.

This era grounded mind–body concepts in physiology and clinical practice, paving the way for integrative medicine.

Today's Leaders & Teachers

- **Dr. Gabor Maté** (*When the Body Says No*): Connects chronic stress, trauma, and suppressed emotions with conditions like autoimmune diseases, cancer, and chronic illness.

- **Dr. Joe Dispenza** (*You Are the Placebo, Becoming Supernatural*): Bridges neuroscience, quantum physics, and meditation—teaching that emotions influence biology and healing.

- **Dr. Bruce Lipton** (*The Biology of Belief*): Stem cell biologist who argues that belief systems and emotions influence gene expression and health (epigenetics).

- **Dr. Bessel van der Kolk** (*The Body Keeps the Score*): A leader in trauma research, showing how unresolved emotional trauma reshapes the nervous system and body, leading to illness.

- **Caroline Myss** (*Anatomy of the Spirit*): Spiritual teacher mapping emotions, energy centers, and illness patterns, building upon both TCM and Christian mysticism.

- **Deborah King** *(Truth Heals: What You Hide Can Hurt You)*, **Inna Segal** (*The Secret Language of Your Body: The Essential Guide to Health and Wellness*), **Isabelle Benarous** *(the Bio-Breakthrough: Decode Your Illness and Heal Your Life)*, and other holistic healers: Expand on Louise Hay's work by linking body symptoms to emotions and offering energetic healing modalities.

From Ayurvedic sages to New Thought philosophers, early psychosomatic researchers to modern clinicians and inspirational teachers, the mind–body–spirit paradigm provides a living legacy. Today's integrative health approaches combining meditation, nutrition, psychotherapy, energy medicine, and conventional care stand on the shoulders of these diverse pioneers. What unites them is a simple, profound recognition that the mind and spirit are not separate from the body. Our thoughts, emotions, and spiritual awareness shape the terrain of health, offering every person the possibility of more profound healing and vitality.

Chapter 21
The Emotional Blueprint of Disease

How Feelings Shape the Body, Mind, and Soul

In *Radiant Wellness*, we explore the interconnectedness of body, mind, and spirit—and nowhere is this connection more profound than in the relationship between our emotions and physical health. While modern medicine often separates the body from the mind, holistic principles have long understood that emotions are not intangible forces floating outside of biology; they are biochemical and energetic messengers influencing every cell in the human body.

Today, a growing number of physicians, neuroscientists, and energy healers are re-examining what ancient wisdom has taught for millennia: that suppressed or unprocessed emotions can distort the body's energy flow, weaken immunity, and create conditions ripe for disease.

Understanding the Energy of Emotion

Every emotion carries a unique vibrational frequency. Love, gratitude, and joy vibrate at higher frequencies that expand our energy field and promote healing. Fear, anger, guilt, and grief vibrate at lower frequencies that contract and stagnate the body's energetic systems.

When emotions are felt, expressed, and released, they flow through us harmlessly. But when they are suppressed—whether due to trauma, denial, or fear of judgment—they create energetic "imprints" in the body's biofield. Over time, these imprints may manifest as physical symptoms or chronic illness.

This concept aligns with both energy medicine and psychoneuroimmunology. The latter shows that emotional stress alters hormone levels, weakens immune defense, and increases inflammation. Meanwhile, energy medicine teaches that the same emotional frequencies distort the flow of Qi (life force), or Prana, producing blockages that correspond to organ imbalances.

Emotions and the Organs: An Introduction to Traditional Chinese Medicine (TCM)

Is there a correlation between our emotions and our organs? Do our organs actually *store* our emotions, that causing dis-ease? According to modern biomedical science, this theory does *not* support the idea that organs "store" emotions in the literal sense (e.g., the liver holding anger). Emotions are understood as emergent from complex interactions of brain, nervous system, hormones, and bodily feedback loops (e.g., the gut–brain axis), not as tied to one discrete organ. Some more recent integrative or psychosomatic medicine approaches acknowledge that emotional states can affect organ *function* (e.g., chronic stress affecting liver metabolism), but that is very different from a one-to-one literal storage. Then, where did the organ theory emerge? Which theory is true - modern science, ancient wisdom, or both?

In our daily rush through life, we often treat emotions as something happening "up here" (in the mind) as fleeting mental states; and organs as something happening "down there" (in the body). However, traditional Chinese medicine (TCM) teaches that this separation is an illusion. Emotions and organs are intimately connected: shifts in how we feel ripple through our Qi (pronounced chee), or vital energy, potentially affecting organ health over time.

Modern science echoes this by showing how stress, grief, or fear alters hormones, immunity, and digestion. Together, these perspectives reveal a profound truth: emotional balance is a foundation of physical health. When we learn to tune into these connections, we gain access to an early warning system within our bodies—one that guides us toward healing before disease takes root.

In TCM, Yin and Yang are complementary forces of balance. Yin is stillness, rest, and deep introspection; Yang is activity, movement, and expression. Emotionally speaking, too much Yang may show up as agitation, restlessness, or over-excitement; an excess of Yin might present as withdrawal, lethargy, or emotional numbness. When yin and yang are balanced, emotions move naturally without overwhelming the organs or Qi pathways (also known as meridians).

Liver & Anger: The Liver governs the smooth flow of Qi and blood throughout the body, making it central to all movement, flexibility, and adaptation. It's also the organ most tied to anger, resentment, and frustration. In an imbalanced pattern, this forms repressed or explosive anger leading to Liver Qi stagnation. When Qi fails to move smoothly, symptoms like tension, headaches, menstrual cramps, digestive upset, and irritability appear. Anger can push Qi upward too aggressively, manifesting as hypertension, dizziness, or insomnia. A balanced liver demonstrates emotional flexibility, patience, and assertiveness rather than aggression.

Heart & Joy: In TCM, the heart is more than a pump—it houses *Shen*, the spirit or mind. Joy is its natural emotion. Yet too much excitement scatters the heart's energy, while too little leaves one in depression or flat affect. Excess joy or mania tends to scatter Heart Qi, manifesting as agitation, insomnia, palpitations, or restlessness. Deficiency or lack of joy leads to dullness, emotional withdrawal, or depressive states. Balanced heart energy provides inner peace, warmth, clarity, and emotional presence.

Spleen & Worry (Pensiveness): The spleen in TCM transforms food into Qi and blood; it is the engine of nourishment and thought. Worry, obsessive thinking, and overanalysis burden it. Excess worry and overthinking lead to Spleen Qi deficiency, manifesting as poor appetite, bloating, diarrhea, fatigue, brain fog, or weak muscles. Qi stagnation in this area can knot the flow of Qi, causing tightness in the chest or digestive discomfort. A fully balanced spleen can provide mental clarity, stable mood, good digestion, and reliable energy.

Lungs & Sadness (Grief): The lungs govern breath, immunity, and our capacity to let go. Their emotional partner is sadness or grief. Prolonged sorrow weakens Lung Qi. Chronic grief or sadness reduces Lung Qi, causing fatigue, frequent colds, shallow breathing, and emotional withdrawal. Over-suppressed grief or the inability to express sorrow may lead to stagnation, heaviness, or difficulty catching one's breath. Balanced Lung Qi offers emotional release (healthy crying), openness, and resilience.

Kidneys & Fear: The kidneys are the root of life energy (Jing), governing growth, reproduction, and willpower. Chronic fear, insecurity, or terror depletes Kidney Qi. Fear and chronic anxiety cause Qi to withdraw, leading to signs like lower-back pain, urinary issues, fatigue, weak bones, and low will. Extreme fear can cause Qi to descend too deeply, manifesting as weakness or collapse. Balanced kidneys produce courage, determination, groundedness, and a steady will.

Organ Transplant Recipients

An interesting side note demonstrating that organs may store emotions comes from organ transplant recipients. Over the years, many interesting reports and case studies suggest that organs are much more than a mere component of the body that performs a function. These reports discuss transplant recipients who have reported changes in preferences, emotions, behaviors, and even memories that they or others feel resemble characteristics of their organ donor(s). Some have observed a change in food preferences, new emotional tendencies or moods, new aversions or fears, changes in artistic or musical tastes, and even occasional purported "memories" or intuitive feelings associated with the donor. In the research literature, a recent survey-based study in a MDPI medical journal found that 89% of organ transplant recipients noted some change in their personality or preferences post-transplant. Another narrative study published in PubMed reported on heart transplant recipients, exploring how some observed preferences, emotions, or memory resemblances to donors, invoking concepts of *heart memory*. Other papers contribute to the transfer of traits to *cellular memory*.

The Three Stages of Emotional Imbalance

This concept is a modern integrative summary that blends ancient medicine, psychosomatic medicine, mind-body medicine, energy medicine, and biofield teachings into a clear format. It's often used in holistic wellness, energy psychology, and metaphysical healing literature to describe how subtle emotional disharmony evolves into physical symptoms if left unresolved.

- **Energetic Disturbance** – Emotional suppression disrupts the body's energy flow, even before symptoms appear.

- **Functional Disharmony** – Hormonal, neurological, or digestive imbalances arise, often accompanied by fatigue, tension, or mild pain.

- **Physical Manifestation** – When left unaddressed, the energy crystallizes into a diagnosable illness or chronic disease pattern.

In this model, disease is not the body's enemy—it is a message, asking us to address emotional, mental, or energetic wounds that have gone unheard.

The Science of Emotion and Biochemistry

Modern neuroscience confirms what ancient systems observed intuitively. The limbic system, the emotional center of the brain, communicates directly with the hypothalamus and pituitary glands, which regulate hormones, metabolism, and immunity.

Chronic emotional stress keeps the body in a "fight-or-flight" state, flooding it with cortisol and adrenaline, which suppress immunity and increase inflammation. Conversely, positive emotions trigger the release of oxytocin, serotonin, and endorphins, as hormones that enhance and repair immunity, and longevity.

While science may not declare that "emotions create disease," research continues to show that emotions influence the onset, progression, and recovery of nearly all chronic illnesses, from heart disease and autoimmune disorders to cancer. Although the language may not be the same, the message echoes this interplay. Emotional states modulate hormonal balance (e.g., cortisol in stress), autonomic nervous system tone (the sympathetic-parasympathetic balance), and immune function. For example, chronic stress weakens digestion, alters gut permeability, and suppresses immunity—phenomena that map quite naturally onto the TCM notion of a Spleen or Lung imbalance.

The one thing that is common ground is that chronic stress has the ability to wreak havoc on our physical and mental health. Our emotions are not enemies to be suppressed; they are messengers guiding us back to balance. By learning the language of your body—how anger, grief, fear, worry, or joy manifest—you can intervene early, restore harmony, and strengthen vitality.

Chapter 22
Understanding Chronic Stress

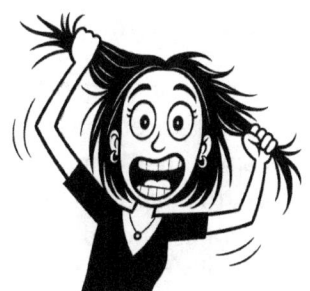

Stress is more than just how you feel – it's a full-body chemical event that can either protect you or quietly dismantle your health from the inside out. Designed as a short-term survival mechanism, the stress response was never meant to be a lifestyle. Yet in our modern world, constant pressure, overstimulation, and emotional strain keep our bodies locked in fight-or-flight mode. Cortisol and adrenaline surge, blood pressure rises, digestion slows, and inflammation spreads. Over time, this biological alarm system, meant to save us, begins to sabotage us, draining our energy, aging our cells, and disrupting the body's natural rhythm of repair. The good news is that stress is not inevitable; it's a signal. When you learn to listen, regulate, and restore balance, calm becomes your greatest medicine and vitality your natural state.

Not to sound like a downer, but there is no way to sugarcoat this: Stress is no longer just a personal burden, it's a silent global pandemic. Around the world, 30–50% of people in 77 countries report experiencing significant psychological stress. In the U.S. alone, the Gallup poll states that 49% of adults say they frequently feel stressed — the highest level recorded in decades. Studies also show that 83% of U.S. workers suffer from work-related stress, and occupational stress contributes to 120,000 deaths annually in this country. Stress has been called "the health epidemic of the 21st century" by global experts.

Let's get to the root causes of our stress so we can create some inner calm. Our work situations tend to be at the forefront, whether we are unhappy with what we are doing, facing stressful work deadlines, or dealing with negative or backstabbing coworkers. Other contributing factors are receiving upsetting news, not feeling safe, political and economic situations, being too busy, caring for a sick or elderly parent, being overwhelmed and overworked, financial woes, and arguments with our spouse or children, all of which contribute to our mental state. Suffering from chronic stress can affect every organ in the body and cause numerous physical problems through the release of a cascade of hormones.

When faced with challenges, the brain triggers the fight-or-flight response, which starts with the release of adrenaline, instantly causing a rise in blood pressure, muscle tension, breathing, heart rate, blood sugar, and slowed digestion. In addition, the hypothalamus-pituitary-adrenal (HPA) axis releases additional hormones, including cortisol, which is released in high amounts during stressful situations. Cortisol directs energy away from processes that are not urgent, such as wound healing and immune system functioning. In other words, stress disrupts the entire body from functioning correctly.

Some of the common health problems caused or exacerbated by stress are digestive problems, heart disease, pain, poor immune health, infections, the recurrence of dormant viruses, sleep disturbances, depression, weight gain, reproductive issues, loss of libido, anxiety, autoimmune diseases, memory issues, and cancer. Stress keeps our bodies in an acidic state. We may be eating a healthy diet full of alkaline foods, but our bodies will be acidic if we are constantly stressed. Emotional stress also causes oxidative stress within the body. This means that it produces free radicals, known to be involved in various diseases, including atherosclerosis (plaque deposits in coronary arteries), kidney disease, Parkinson's disease, and Alzheimer's disease. It also accelerates aging at the cellular level. It is easy to tell a person's emotional state by looking at their faces. Stress makes us look years older than we are. To make the problem worse, people often use prescription medications, drugs, and alcohol to ease the distress, causing even more acidity in the body. We can also blame stress for promoting the overeating of unhealthy comfort foods, which further contributes to poor health and harmful side effects. A lethal double-whammy!

We all face stress as a part of life, but emotional stress is not caused by our actual problems but by the way in which we interpret and react to the situations we encounter. How we respond to stress can directly impact our health by lowering immune function and creating exhaustion.

Personality Types. Mental health professionals believe personality plays a significant role in how we perceive stressful situations. High-strung and overly emotional people tend to react poorly to unfavorable circumstances. Type A personalities tend to be rushed, ambitious, time-conscious, and driven. Studies suggest these traits, if not properly managed, can create stress-related illnesses. In contrast, the Type B personality is a much more relaxed, less time-conscious, driven person. In contrast, Type B personalities generally view things more adaptively. They are better able to put things into perspective and think through how they will deal with situations, tending to be less stress prone. Some studies show that gender plays a role, possibly due to hormones, claiming women tend to become more stressed out and emotional than men.

Inherited Stress. Recent research suggests that our response to stress could be influenced by our experiences in the womb. Scientists have been studying correlations between how the creation of maternal stress creates high levels of cortisol in the body during pregnancy could affect the development of the baby. According to the research, if a mother has high cortisol levels, the fetus will have similarly high levels. As a result, this exposure could affect the level of receptors for stress-related substances in the baby's brain, making them more susceptible to stressors later in life (Thanks, Mom!).

Regardless, the key here is not to change our personality or who we are. Those who are more susceptible to stress are not doomed. Learning to manage our stress is vital to our health. The goal is to notice when we feel stressed. Start by slowing down, taking a brief time-out, and slowly inhale a few deep breaths throughout the day. Try to pinpoint the cause of the stress. At times, you may find that it's a cascade of things trickling down. Think yourself through it. Is it something you can change or something that you need to accept? With a little work, we can train our mindset to see things in a new light. This mind frame is not learned overnight. However, with conscious effort, we can greatly improve by doing a few things to help ease the daily stress we may be experiencing.

Create a Sacred Environment. Our homes should be our castle and a place of refuge. However, some of the most obvious situations such as incessant noise, chaos, racing thoughts, and problems keep us in constant turmoil. The utmost goal is to experience peace in any environment, even if it is loud, disruptive, or annoying. However, while we are in training (which we all are throughout our existence), rearranging our environments to create a calming vibe can certainly help. For instance, let's compare two different scenarios.

Scenario #1: You are in your house. The kids are screaming, the dog is barking, the gardeners are blowing their leaf blowers, the television is blaring in one room and loud rock music is pounding through a different room. There is clutter everywhere, and dirty dishes are piling up in the sink. A distinct odor of garbage fills the air.

Scenario #2: You are in your house. It is quiet, with relaxing instrumental piano music piped in throughout. A cool breeze is finding its way in through the open window, along with the sound of the trickling brook from the fountain. The relaxing aroma of lavender fills the air. The sun is peeking through the clouds, filling your room with a beautiful, bright light.

Can you feel your energy shift once you were visiting the second scenario? Granted, Scenario #1 is more than likely the norm in our modern world. If this is the case for you, find an area cut off from the noise to make a sacred space, even if it is just your bedroom. Spend time each day in a positive environment, both for work and relaxation, where you can just relax or sit in silence.

Breathwork. Incorporating breathwork exercises as part of a daily ritual is thought to positively influence our spiritual, mental, emotional, and physical health. Breathwork is a highly effective way to activate your body's parasympathetic nervous system which helps to de-stress and reset the nervous system. When we take slow, deep breaths, our brain receives signals to relax and disengage from the stress response. This process reduces tension and enhances oxygen flow throughout our body, promoting better cellular function and mental clarity. It fosters mindfulness, grounding us in the present moment and reducing the tendency to dwell on past events or worry about the future. The best part is everybody can do it and benefit from it. All you need are your lungs. There are numerous articles and videos describing different breathwork techniques. With a bit of research, you will soon be able to determine what would work best for you.

My favorite for simplicity is what is referred to as the Box (or Square) Breathing or 4-4-4-4. You simply sit, stand, or lie down comfortably, and then inhale through the nose for four counts, hold your breath for four counts, exhale through the mouth for the duration of four counts, and finally, wait again for four counts before your next inhale.

The most prominent benefit of Box Breathing is its ability to instantly provide calming relaxation within just a few minutes. This technique can be done at any time of the day. It helps people fall asleep sooner, lowers blood pressure, combats anxiety and panic, controls moments of hyperventilation, and increases concentration and focus.

Tapping. Tapping, also known as the emotional freedom technique (EFT), is a simple technique founded by Gary Craig. In this technique, you gently tap specific meridian points of your body while focusing on distressing thoughts or emotions. It has been clinically proven to manage stress, reduce cortisol levels, improve anxiety, and treat PTSD. Many books, classes, and videos teach this technique. A good place to start is to visit Gary's website at www.palaceofpossibilities.com to watch his informative intro video.

HeartMath. HeartMath is a science-based app that uses heart rate variability (HRV) to help users regulate their emotions and behaviors to reduce stress through guided meditation and biofeedback to balance the nervous system and adrenal function. Studies conducted with over 14,000 people have shown long-lasting improvements in mental and emotional well-being in just 6-9 weeks. Visit www.HeartMath.com for details.

Exercise. Exercise helps to raise the production of our brain's feel-good neurotransmitters, called endorphins. Although this function is often referred to as a runner's high, any aerobic activity, such as jumping jacks or a brisk walk, can contribute to this same feeling. There are times, such as being up against a serious deadline, when you may think taking a time-out would be impossible. However, this may be the time you need it the most. The good news is that studies show that just five minutes of exercise can produce anti-anxiety effects, calm the mind, and allow you to work more effectively. This time-out concept relates to Stephen Covey's concept of *sharpening the saw*. In other words, taking a mini break to renew and refresh your panicked emotional state will allow you to return stronger, clearer, and calmer, completing the task sooner with more efficiency.

Gratitude. Did you know it's impossible to experience stress and gratitude simultaneously? Changing our mindset from victim mode to practicing gratitude can help reduce anxiety by shifting focus to positive aspects of life, promoting relaxation, and boosting overall well-being. Focusing on what we're grateful for can trigger the release of neurotransmitters like dopamine and serotonin, which can help calm our nervous system and reduce anxiety. Laughing will also do the same, however being in a constant state of gratitude is much easier by simply making a conscious effort to remember to appreciate the small things in our day.

An Old-Fashioned Bubble Bath. The *Calgon, take me away,* slogan had some merit after all. Relaxing in a bathtub full of hot water can be therapeutic physically, emotionally, and spiritually. Hot water helps increase our blood flow to the skin. The temperature of the bath can also improve our breathing. Baths are an excellent way to relax, relieve everyday stressors, and feel pampered. Not only does it feel good to have some time to ourselves, but submergence in water helps calm the nervous system, reduce stress and anxiety levels in the body, and improve our mood. Warm baths can stimulate the production of serotonin, the chemical in the brain associated with happiness. So, whenever that feeling of unease creeps up, or if you are seeking refuge from a long, stressful day, a nice warm bubble bath may be just what the doctor ordered. One suggestion is to look for organic bubble bath products. Add Epsom salts and calming lavender essential oil for an extra health bonus.

Aromatherapy. Aromatherapy can help reduce stress and anxiety, improve mood, and promote better sleep by calming the nervous system. People who respond well to scents could benefit from using a diffuser. I recommend the following oils for calming: 1) Lavender can promote relaxation and improve sleep quality in people with insomnia, 2) Ylang-ylang can help decrease blood pressure and create a relaxing effect, 3) Bergamot can stimulate feelings of joy and optimism and provide relief from anxiety and depression, 4) Chamomile can reduce anxiety and improve sleep, and 5) Clary sage can decrease cortisol levels, the hormone responsible for stress.

Trauma. Emotions, mindset, negativity, programming, and fearful thinking can all contribute to chronic stress that can be reversed with self-reflection and journaling. These patterns did not appear overnight but through a lifetime of experience of traumatic events, both large and small.

Gadgets. If you like trying small, innovative gadgets, you may want to explore *truVaga*. It is a vagus nerve stimulator that helps your body manage its fight-or-flight response with just a 2-minute session, day or night. It claims to relieve stress, improve sleep, and enhance clarity. There is also a nice wearable product to experiment with called *Apollo* that comes with a 30-day free trial.

Supplementation. Supplementation can provide calming for the nervous system while nourishing the adrenals. When life keeps us in constant motion, our nervous system often forgets what peace feels like. Over time, stress hormones like cortisol stay elevated, leaving us tired yet wired, anxious, or unable to fully rest. Nature has provided us with a pharmacy of herbs and nutrients that gently guide the body back to balance, soothing the mind, calming the adrenals, and restoring harmony to the entire system.

Among the most powerful are the *adaptogens*—herbs that help the body adapt to stress and build resilience. Ashwagandha is one of the most popular herbs and used in many stress formulations. It helps lower cortisol levels, ease anxiety, and brings the endocrine system into balance. Clinical studies show it can reduce stress markers by nearly a third, and its grounding energy makes it ideal for those who feel depleted or overwhelmed.

Rhodiola rosea offers a more uplifting form of support. Rather than simply sedating the nervous system, it sharpens mental clarity and stabilizes energy by balancing cortisol rhythms. It's often chosen by those who experience fatigue, low motivation, or burnout.

Holy basil, or *tulsi*, is another adaptogenic herb. In Ayurveda, it's known as the "elixir of life" for its ability to calm the heart and clear the mind. It helps regulate cortisol and blood sugar while gently lifting the mood. Eleuthero, also called Siberian ginseng, strengthens stamina and immune resilience—an excellent ally for those recovering from long periods of stress or illness. And Schisandra, a tonic berry from traditional Chinese medicine, protects the liver, brightens mental focus, and nourishes the adrenals all at once.

While adaptogens build strength from within, the nervine herbs focus on soothing the surface waves of tension and anxiety. Lemon balm is a plant that quiets nervous energy and promotes relaxation without drowsiness. Its gentle citrus aroma alone can ease the mind. Passionflower works a little deeper, slowing racing thoughts and supporting calm focus through its action on GABA, one of the brain's primary calming neurotransmitters. Skullcap is a wonderful companion for the overthinker, relaxing muscular tension while quieting mental chatter.

To complement these plant allies, several nutrients and amino acids can enhance calm from a biochemical level. Magnesium (especially in glycinate or threonate form) is essential for relaxation and supports healthy nerve function. Many people feel its difference within days, especially when taken in the evening. Vitamin C and the B vitamins are vital for adrenal health, as these glands draw heavily on both to make stress hormones. When stress is chronic, they can be quickly depleted, leaving us feeling drained.

L-theanine, a soothing amino acid found naturally in green tea, encourages calm alertness—helping the mind stay centered even during challenging moments. Omega-3 fatty acids from fish or algae oils help regulate inflammation and cortisol release, supporting both mood and cognition. And phosphatidylserine, a compound found in the brain's cell membranes, has been shown to reduce excessive cortisol after stress, improving focus and mental recovery.

HERBS & NUTRIENTS FOR STRESS SUPPORT

HERB OR NUTRIENT	PRIMARY ACTION	BEST FORM
ADAPTOGENS		
Ashwagandha	Lowers cortisol	Capsule
Rhodiola rosea	Improves focus	Capsule
Holy basil	Balances cortisol	Capsule, tea or tincture
Eleuthero	Supports stamina	Capsule
Schisandra	Nourishes adrenals	Capsule
NERVINES		
Lemon balm	Promotes relaxation	Capsule or tea
Passionflower	Quiets mind	Capsule
Valerian	Encourages sleep	Capsule or tincture
Chamomile	Comforts digestion	Capsule or tea
Skullcap	Eases nervous tension	Capsule or tincture
NUTRIENTS		
Magnesium	Supports relaxation	Capsule
Vitamin C & B–complex	Supports adrenal function	Capsule
L-theanine	Promotes calm alertness	Capsule or oil

Chapter 23
Emotional Mastery

The Art of Inner Balance. Emotional mastery is the ability to recognize, understand, and regulate your emotions with awareness and grace. It doesn't mean suppressing how you feel or pretending that negative emotions don't exist. Rather, it's about responding instead of reacting—choosing how to engage with life's challenges from a calm, grounded place rather than from fear or impulsivity. When we master our emotions, we become the conscious creators of our experience rather than victims of circumstance.

At its core, emotional mastery is the art of being centered amid the storm. It's cultivating the awareness that emotions are simply energy in motion—signals guiding us toward what needs healing, releasing, or realignment. Instead of letting emotions control us, we learn to observe them, process them, and use their wisdom to grow.

Why Emotional Mastery Matters. Our emotions directly affect every aspect of our lives—our health, relationships, decisions, and overall energy field. Chronic stress, anger, or fear can disrupt hormonal balance, weaken immunity, and drain vitality. On the other hand, emotions like joy, peace, and love create coherence in the heart and brain, promoting healing and resilience.

Science now confirms what ancient wisdom has long known: emotions alter our biochemistry. Positive emotions can elevate serotonin and endorphins, while prolonged negative emotions can raise cortisol and inflammatory markers. When we master our emotional responses, we not only protect our mental health but also influence our physical well-being at a cellular level.

Just as emotions can make or break our physical health, they can also become the energetic architects of every dimension of our life, shaping our relationships, finances, creativity, intuition, and even our ability to manifest desires. Let's explore a summary of key areas regarding this concept.

Emotions and Relationships. Emotions act as vibrational magnets. We attract people who resonate with our emotional frequency. Unhealed emotions like resentment, fear of abandonment, or shame often create patterns of repeated conflict, codependency, or emotional distance. For example, suppressed anger may draw controlling partners, while unworthiness can lead to one-sided relationships. Healed emotions foster harmony and authenticity. When you process emotions through awareness and self-forgiveness, you naturally attract partners and friends who match your self-respect and emotional maturity.

Emotions and Prosperity. Money is not just a material exchange; it's an energetic mirror of our beliefs and emotions about worth and trust. Fear or scarcity mindset ("I'll never have enough") constricts the flow of opportunities, similar to how tension constricts blood flow in the body. Consequently, one can have a fear of success, fear of failure, etc.

Gratitude and self-worth expand receptivity. The emotion of appreciation literally opens neural pathways linked to creativity and risk-taking, allowing more inspired action toward abundance. Many holistic traditions, from ancient Feng Shui to modern quantum metaphysics, teach that prosperity flows where energy is clear, open, and joyful.

Emotions and Manifestation. Manifestation is not just about affirmations; it's about emotional alignment. In other words, you can say affirmations until you're blue in the face, but if you don't believe you are worthy of the request, the emotional alignment will not match the request. Thoughts create the blueprint, but emotion charges the field. When your emotions are congruent with your desire (e.g., feeling joy *as if it's already real*), your vibrational frequency matches the outcome. Conversely, when fear or doubt dominate, you send mixed signals to the universe, creating delays or blocks.

Science meets spirituality: The HeartMath Institute has shown that coherent heart-brain states, achieved through elevated emotions like gratitude or love, measurably affect electromagnetic fields and influence probability patterns.

Emotions and Happiness. Happiness is not a goal; it's a vibrational state of coherence. Chronic negative emotions like guilt or envy lower our vibrational frequency and trigger stress hormones, hijacking the body's natural joy chemistry. When we regularly express emotions, we release stagnation, the emotional equivalent of detoxing the body. Positive emotions like compassion, awe, and joy release oxytocin, serotonin, and endorphins, reinforcing both physical vitality and a sense of connection.

Integrating Emotional Mastery. True mastery is not avoiding emotion but transmuting it into energy for creation. Here's a holistic framework:

- Recognize – Name the emotion honestly.
- Release – Breathe, cry, move, or write to let it move through you.
- Reframe – Ask, "What is this emotion trying to teach me?"
- Re-align – Choose a new thought or action that matches your desired vibration.

When you live this way, life stops happening *to* you and begins unfolding *through* you.

The following reflections invite you to look within and observe how emotions influence your state of being. Use them as quiet moments of self-inquiry and gentle transformation.

- What emotions most often take control of your day, and what are they trying to teach you?
- When was the last time you paused before reacting—how did that shift the outcome?
- Are there emotions you tend to suppress or avoid? What might happen if you allowed them to surface?
- How might your relationships change if you practiced empathy and curiosity instead of judgment?
- What daily rituals can help you return to inner balance when life feels overwhelming?

Take a few minutes each day to breathe, observe, and realign. Over time, you'll notice that emotional turbulence loses its power and inner peace becomes your natural state. This is emotional mastery in motion: the graceful art of living from the heart.

Throughout this section, we will discuss the various subsections and exercises that will have us oozing with emotional mastery in no time. Be patient with yourself (and others). This is not easy. But before we begin on our lifelong goal of building mastery, we have to do a little clean-up first by building and starting with a strong foundation of self-worth and forgiveness.

Self-Worth. First and foremost, we must understand that our self-worth is not determined by what others think of us. It is not defined by how much money we have in the bank, what car we drive, the size or location of our house, our level of education, where our kids go to school or what they accomplished or do for a living, who we're married to, the people we know, how attractive and fit we are, our popularity, the number of friends or followers we have on social media, or how high up the ladder we are in our careers. Our self-worth is determined by only one thing: That is how *we* value ourselves. Self-worth is the quiet knowing that we are valuable simply because we exist. True self-worth comes from within and recognizing we are inherently worthy and divine beings, deserving of love, respect, and fulfillment.

While self-esteem often fluctuates depending on success or failure, self-worth is constant. It is our unshakable foundation of our inner knowing. When we honor our worth, we no longer seek validation from the outside world; instead, we live from a place of inner confidence and authenticity.

Our sense of worthiness influences every decision we make from the relationships we choose, the opportunities we pursue, even how we treat our bodies. If we subconsciously believe we are "not enough," we may settle for less, sabotage our success, or accept unhealthy dynamics. Conversely, when we know our value, we naturally align with experiences that reflect that truth back to us.

Low self-worth can manifest as people-pleasing, perfectionism, procrastination, or chronic self-criticism. These are often defense mechanisms built over time, rooted in early experiences or cultural conditioning. Yet, the good news is that self-worth can be rebuilt through awareness, compassion, and self-care.

On the energetic level, self-worth sets the vibration for everything we attract. When we radiate worthiness, we magnetize abundance, love, and respect. The universe responds to how we treat ourselves. Believing we are enough is not arrogance but the alignment with our soul's truth.

Self-Worth as the Starting Point of Self-Mastery. Every journey of transformation begins with self-worth. Before we can master our emotions, habits, or consciousness, we must first believe we are *worthy* of healing, peace, and joy. Without this foundation, self-improvement becomes a form of self-rejection, an endless attempt to "fix" what was never broken.

When self-worth is present, we no longer strive to prove our value; we act from it. We make nourishing choices, set healthy boundaries, and invest in our well-being because we know we deserve it. Self-worth anchors us in self-love, and self-love opens the door to self-mastery.

Think of it as the soil in which all growth takes root. You cannot plant the seeds of joy, peace, or empowerment in barren ground. Cultivating self-worth enriches that soil so that every aspect of your personal evolution can flourish.

Building and strengthening your self-worth is a gentle, ongoing process of returning to yourself. It's not about striving to become more, it's about remembering who you already are. There are many ways to strengthen this inner foundation, and each begins with awareness and compassion.

One of the most important steps is to release comparison. The moment we compare our journey to someone else's, we disconnect from our own light. Every soul has a unique path, and what is meant for you will never pass you by. Instead of measuring yourself against others, learn to celebrate their light while nurturing your own.

Another powerful practice is self-compassion. Speak to yourself with patience, understanding, and kindness. When you stumble or fall short, resist the urge to criticize. Growth requires gentleness, not judgment. The way you speak to yourself becomes the tone of your inner world.

To deepen your self-worth, begin to reprogram limiting beliefs that may have taken root long ago. Notice any thoughts that whisper, *"I'm not good enough,"* or *"I don't deserve happiness."* These are not truths as they are simply learned responses from the past. Replace them with empowering affirmations such as, *"I am learning. I am growing. I am worthy of all good things."* Over time, these new beliefs create new neural pathways, shifting your inner dialogue from doubt to confidence.

And finally, remember to celebrate your small wins. Self-worth flourishes when we recognize progress, even baby steps. Each step toward self-honoring, no matter how small, reinforces the belief that you are enough. Take a moment each day to acknowledge your courage, your kindness, or simply your effort to show up for yourself. In doing so, you strengthen the most important relationship you will ever have — the one with you!

"To forgive is to set a prisoner free and to discover that the prisoner was you."
- Lewis B. Smedes

Forgiveness. Any traumatic event in our lives, whether it is a childhood trauma, an unhealthy relationship, emotional or physical abuse, no matter how big or small, gets stored in our subconscious mind in the form of what is called cellular memory. If it isn't addressed and dealt with, it festers into more serious issues in our emotional and physical health. Most traumas in life require clearing by forgiveness. Forgiveness is one of the most profound acts of self-liberation. It is not about condoning another's actions or pretending that pain never occurred. It's about choosing peace over resentment and freeing yourself from the energetic chains that bind you to the past. True forgiveness releases the heavy emotions that keep your heart closed and your energy blocked.

Let's start with the first order of business: Self-Forgiveness. Forgiveness and unconditional love for ourselves. How can we expect others to love and respect us if we cannot love ourselves? One of the primary reasons we suffer this dilemma is because we regret something we once did that was wrong, hurtful, harmful, etc., either to ourselves or another person, that we haven't resolved yet. We may be holding guilt, shame, embarrassment, remorse, etc. Holding these low vibrational energies simply has to go! Starting today. To be human is to make mistakes. The past is just that. We cannot go back in time with the consciousness we have right now. In other words, who we are today is not who we were yesterday. All that has happened to us in the past makes us who we are today. Appreciate you have this moment to put this issue to rest. Take the time to forgive yourself. Bless it and release it from your consciousness. Until this step is complete, you need not continue with the rest.

Holding on to anger, betrayal, or guilt is like drinking poison and expecting the other person to suffer. It keeps the body in a constant state of tension, elevates stress hormones, and diminishes vitality. On a spiritual level, unforgiveness lowers our vibration and clouds our ability to see life through the lens of love. Forgiveness, on the other hand, restores flow, harmony, and coherence within the body, mind, and soul.

Self-mastery begins with inner peace, and forgiveness is the key that unlocks it. Before we can rise into higher states of awareness, we must clear the emotional weight that keeps us anchored in the past. Resentment, shame, and self-blame act like emotional toxins that cloud clarity, distort perception, and prevent us from aligning with our higher self.

To reiterate, forgiving others is not about forgetting, excusing, or minimizing what happened. It's about understanding that holding on to bitterness only prolongs our suffering. Everyone acts from their level of consciousness at the time. Recognizing this doesn't make their actions right — it simply allows us to release the energetic charge that keeps us tethered to their behavior. When we choose forgiveness, we are declaring that, *"I will no longer allow this pain to define me."* Forgiveness is not weakness; it is strength of the highest order. It is the courageous act of choosing love over fear.

When you forgive, you are not saying, *"What you did is okay."* You are saying, *"I am ready to heal."* You stop replaying the egoic mind and open the space for new experiences to enter. Forgiveness dissolves the energetic cords that bind you to pain and replaces them with compassion and understanding.

You'll know you've truly forgiven when you can think of the situation without emotional intensity and when peace replaces pain. Sometimes, this takes time and layers of healing, but every small release brings more lightness and freedom.

How to Forgive – Practical Paths to Letting Go. Forgiving and letting go can look differently to different people. It's important to find a method that feels authentic for you. You many need more than one method until you feel that release that brings you the peace that sets you free. One of the most healing ways to forgive is to give your feelings a voice. Begin by writing a heartfelt letter you'll never send — a private space to express every emotion, truth, or regret you've held inside. Let the words flow freely without judgment or censoring. If the person is still alive and it feels right in your heart, you may choose to offer a genuine apology or extend forgiveness in person. Speak from authenticity, not blame. You might say something like, *"I've been holding on to pain from our past, and I'm ready to release it. I forgive you for your part in it, and I hope you can forgive me for mine."* The goal isn't to reopen wounds but to restore peace within yourself. If the person is no longer living, find a quiet, sacred space where you won't be interrupted and speak to their photograph or simply to their spirit. Share what needs to be said. Explain how they made you feel and how you were hurt and betrayed by their actions. Tell them you know they did not have the consciousness to understand how it would have affected you and that you are now releasing the situation to the universe/God.

Another effective healing method for some is an ancient Hawaiian practice called Ho'oponopono (pronounced ho-oh-pono-pono), method for reconciliation and inner cleansing. Its simplicity makes it incredibly powerful. You repeat four phrases with presence and sincerity, directing them toward the person or situation in need of healing, or toward yourself. It goes like this: "I'm sorry. Please forgive me. Thank you. I love you." Each phrase holds a vibrational frequency that softens resistance and restores harmony. *I'm sorry* acknowledges awareness of harm or imbalance. *Please forgive me* opens the heart to release. T*hank you* shifts energy toward gratitude. *I love you* reconnects you with divine compassion. It may feel strange at first, but the repetition creates healing energy. Studies on heart-brain coherence and forgiveness meditation show reduced stress and improved emotional resilience when these phrases are practiced regularly.

Begin to notice something miraculous starts to happen within. The emotional debris that once clouded your heart begins to lift, and energy starts to move freely again — like sunlight breaking through after a long storm. The body softens, the breath deepens, and the heart returns to its natural rhythm of coherence and vitality. This renewed flow of energy is not just emotional; it's physical, spiritual, and cellular. It's as though the very essence of life starts to hum again, resonating with peace instead of pain. Forgiveness doesn't erase what happened — it transforms the way it lives within you. In that transformation, your energy becomes lighter, clearer, and more aligned with love. And it is from this liberated space that the true *energy of release* can emerge — the sacred process of returning to wholeness.

Chapter 24
Cultivating Happiness & Joy

Happiness and joy may seem like interchangeable emotions, but they stem from very different roots. Happiness often depends on external circumstances such as a promotion, a sunny day, meeting a close friend for lunch, or cashing in on a winning lottery ticket. It's the emotional response to something going right in our world. Joy, on the other hand, is deeper and more lasting. It's the quiet, soulful contentment that arises from within that persists even when life is uncertain. Joy doesn't wait for everything to be perfect; it's the light that shines despite what's happening around us. Here is where we can shine. When life presents challenges, we can either sink into self-pity or rise into the possibility of transforming obstacles into opportunities for growth.

From a scientific standpoint, cultivating happiness and joy is far more than a feel-good pursuit; it's a vital component of whole-body health and longevity. Positive emotions have been shown to lower cortisol, reduce inflammation, and strengthen the immune system. They regulate heart rhythm, improve sleep, and even enhance cellular repair. Joy literally changes our biochemistry, shifting us from stress-based living to vitality-based thriving.

Spiritually, joy aligns our vibration with the energy of creation itself. When we live in joy, we become magnetic to synchronicities, opportunities, and loving connections. It's as if the universe begins to conspire with us for our highest good. Happiness opens the door, but joy invites us to stay there and live from a place of gratitude, peace, and presence.

Cultivating happiness and joy isn't about denying life's challenges; it's about training the mind and heart to see beauty even in the midst of them. We can nurture this state through mindfulness, gratitude practices, laughter, creative expression, acts of kindness, spending time in nature, and surrounding ourselves with uplifting people. Each of these small choices helps us tune in to a higher frequency where contentment, meaning, and lightness naturally reside. Ultimately, happiness and joy are not destinations, but daily practices and gentle reminders that wellness is not just about the body's vitality, but the soul's ability to shine through every experience.

Why We Struggle to Live Joyfully: If joy is our natural state, why do so many people find it elusive? Often, it's not that joy has left us—It's that our joy is being blocked by the layers of fear, conditioning, and emotional residue that have clouded our ability to feel it. True joy is always within reach, but several common barriers can dull its light.

- **Emotional Baggage and Unhealed Wounds.** Past pain, disappointment, or trauma can weigh heavily on the heart. When emotions remain unprocessed, they linger in the subconscious, shaping our perceptions and reactions. We may unconsciously guard ourselves from new experiences of joy out of fear of being hurt again. Healing begins when we allow ourselves to feel, release, and forgive—clearing space for joy to return.

- **Living in Survival Mode.** Modern life keeps many people locked in a state of chronic stress. When the body is in "fight-or-flight," the nervous system prioritizes survival over serenity. High cortisol levels, lack of rest, and constant stimulation make it nearly impossible to access feelings of peace or happiness. Joy requires safety, relaxation, and presence.

- **Attachment to External Validation.** When our happiness depends on external conditions such as approval, success, relationships, or material things, joy becomes fragile and fleeting. We chase the next thing that promises fulfillment, only to feel empty again once it's achieved. Joy blossoms when we detach from outcomes and cultivate inner satisfaction independent of circumstances.

- **Negative Thinking and Comparison.** The mind can be a powerful ally or a relentless critic. Dwelling on what's wrong, replaying old stories, or comparing ourselves to others lowers our vibration. These thought patterns disconnect us from gratitude—the very frequency where joy resides. Shifting to appreciation and self-compassion restores balance and emotional clarity.

- **Lack of Connection or Purpose.** Humans are wired for connection and meaning. When we feel isolated, purposeless, or disconnected from something greater than ourselves, joy naturally fades. Joy thrives when we feel we belong, when we contribute, and when our daily actions align with our values and soul's calling.

- **Resistance to the Present Moment.** Much of our suffering arises from living in the past or worrying about the future. Joy can only exist in the *now*. When we surrender to the present—even if it's imperfect—we rediscover life's simple pleasures: a deep breath, sunlight on the skin, laughter with a friend. Presence opens the gateway to joy.

- **Being out of Alignment.** When we're not living the life our soul truly desires, we will lack joy. Joy is a kind of an inner compass; when we feel it, it's often a sign that we're walking our authentic path. When it disappears, it may be the soul's quiet way of saying, *"This isn't where I'm meant to be."*

The following reflections are offered as gentle invitations to pause, look within, and notice where joy might be lacking in our lives. Use them for contemplation, self-inquiry, or journaling your way back to alignment and joy.

What Would You Do IF . . . What would you be doing in your life if money were not an issue? Recently, the Lottery jackpot reached an inconceivable amount—well over a billion dollars. People from all walks of life, from young to old, were lining up to purchase their tickets for the chance to become the latest billionaire and claim unlimited happiness in their lives. It was interesting to observe. I often pondered what each person would do if they woke up one day to find they were instantly wealthy beyond their dreams. I wondered if they even knew.

I decided to have some fun with this topic. I surveyed a handful of acquaintances to learn what they would do if they won the jackpot. Without hesitation, nearly everyone had grandiose visions. Often, couples had dreams that were opposite from their mates. The bottom line is that everyone would be doing something other than what they are presently doing. What I found interesting was that everybody I asked was not even dabbling in or with their interests or dreams, even in the smallest way. What limiting beliefs or excuses hold us back from creating the best life we can dream of? Lack of funds? Waiting for an "event" to happen first? Waiting for the last kid to get through high school, college, etc.? Are you convinced that dreams are just a fairytale? Fear of change? Fear of failure?

While winning the lotto would certainly be nice, statistics tell us that we have approximately 1 in 13.98 million chances that our winning numbers will be drawn. So, what other things can we do to set our dreams into motion?

What excites us? When we do what we love, our light shines. When we awaken each morning with purpose, something within us shifts. Our energy rises, our minds clear, and our hearts open to a quiet sense of joy. Purpose gives rhythm and meaning to life. Ask yourself right now: If you had the ability to make every day the *best* day of your life, what would that day look like? Whether you are sick, broke, or burdened with responsibilities, allow yourself to take this mental break. Imagine yourself as free as a bird with no issues whatsoever and let's continue with a short visualization technique.

> Funny, but true...
> One Sunday, a middle-aged man in need of financial assistance walks into a church and kneels at the altar and begins to pray to God, stating that he has many unpaid bills and asks to win the lottery. After he is done praying, he gets up and walks out.
>
> The following Sunday he goes back to the same church and pleads with God through his prayers to let him win the lottery so that he can pay these past-due bills.
>
> The third Sunday comes around and the man enters the church very upset and close to tears. He kneels at the alter and asks God why he is doing this to him and say's that he has asked to win the lottery for three weeks now and nothing. Suddenly there came a loud bang of thunder and God spoke, "Please! At least meet me halfway and buy a lottery ticket!"

Visualization Exercise. Visualization techniques are not just daydreaming—they're scientifically proven to rewire the brain and thought patterns and help you manifest what you want in life (and it's fun, too!). Have you ever heard the saying that the universe can't give you what you want if it doesn't know what it is?

On your computer or in a notebook, you will become the architect of your surroundings and the screenwriter of your ideal life. Remove all limitations from your energy field. Let your imagination flow. The sky is the limit! Without overthinking it, start scribbling out your dream life. The more details you provide, the better. Note: Winning the lottery is not allowed in this visualization.

In your vision, starting with the moment you wake up, look around your room. Describe what it looks like. What does your bed feel like? What do you see outside your window? Who (if anyone) is lying beside you? Where do you live? Do you live in a beach house? A mansion? In the country? On a yacht? In a treehouse in Costa Rica? Describe your surroundings or the town or island where you live. What is the temperature outside? Is there an aroma in the air? What are your neighbors like? Do you have a job that you love? Do you drive to a destination, or do you work from your home? Do you work at all? Describe your friends. What activities will you be doing on this day and night? What will you wear? How will you get there? Are you feeling pain-free? Healthy? Abundant? Carefree? Blissful? Loved? Who do you encounter along the way? What do you eat or drink? Who are you socializing with? Is there music playing in the background?

Continue this exercise until you aren't able to think of a single thing you still desire. When you are finished, write at the bottom of your story, "*This, or something better, is now manifesting for me and my highest good*". It is always best to add, *or "something better"* because sometimes we cannot comprehend all the good that is available to us, and the universe may have something bigger and better in the works.

Vision Boards. Visual people may get more benefit from creating a vision board. A vision board is a tool used for visualization and goal setting, featuring a collage of images, words, and affirmations from magazines, photos, drawings, quotes, and other visuals that resonate with your goals and aspirations, representing the things you want to manifest. Creating a visual representation of your goals and desires helps clarify your intentions and keeps them at the forefront of your mind. Think of it as a business plan and blueprint for bringing your dreams to life.

Now that you have visualized your ideal life, list five things that you can do to set it in motion. It doesn't need to be anything extravagant or costly like putting a down payment on a plot of land (although that would be a great step if it were available to you). It can be something like researching available rentals in (name of dream town), checking online for jobs in (name of city), taking a class to learn something that can help create your vision, volunteering at a place that can improve your skills, etc. You get the point. Doing nothing creates stagnation. Setting dreams in motion creates momentum. It offers a mindset that, *yeah, just maybe, I can pull this off.* Creating dreams puts spark and purpose back into our lives.

Affirmations. We have all heard the sayings, *what you think you become*, or *where your attention goes, the energy flows*. However, there is more to this than quotes. Research in neuroscience has shown that affirmations can activate specific brain regions associated with self-processing and emotional regulation. Studies using MRI scans have shown that affirmations stimulate the ventromedial prefrontal cortex, reinforcing positive self-identity. This activation helps reshape negative thought patterns and promotes a more optimistic outlook. In a nutshell, as long as chronic negative emotions and limiting beliefs are lurking in our energy field, we will be operating in low vibrational energy (fear and lack). Being in a negative state will attract more of the same. In order to change our energy into a more radiant and flourishing environment, we need to acknowledge our emotions and bring them out into the light so that we can release the emotions that no longer serve us and replace them with what we desire out of life. This rewires our brain and is accomplished through intentions and affirmations. An intention is a spark of consciousness that contains the seed form of that which we aim to create. Co-creating what we truly desire brings fulfillment, a sense of purpose, and the joy of living. The mind is a powerful tool if we decide to use it as one.

The subconscious mind cannot tell the difference between reality and imagination. Therefore, regularly repeating affirming statements leads to convincing our mind that the visions are fact, leading to us believing we can do it. When we realize and release our intentions into our conscious and subconscious energy fields, we make way for them to manifest and flourish. Trust and know the Universe/Spirit/God has your back. You are worthy of all the wonders life has to offer and the complete fulfillment of all your desires.

Creating affirmations is quite easy. However, you can't just create them and set them aside. They need to be worked with and ingrained into your consciousness. When creating your affirmations, remember to always word them with positivity. For example, you wouldn't want to word an affirmation such as "I disassociate myself from negative people." Your subconscious hears the words negative people and that's what you may get. A correctly written affirmation would be "I attract positive and loving people into my life." Words are energy and the way they are used matters. As a matter of fact, not long ago, I was speaking to a practitioner. I explained to him that my digestion is messed up. He immediately corrected me and said you may want to rephrase that as *My digestion could use some improvement.* I was grateful for the reminder.

Be creative with your affirmations. Here are some ideas that can help start the process:

- My soul is ready to live the life of my dreams.
- I deserve all that life has to offer.
- I have the skills and abilities to achieve all that I desire.
- I believe in myself and can achieve my goals.
- I view all situations in my life as opportunities for growth.
- I trust myself and follow my instincts.
- I am becoming a better version of myself each day.
- I am grateful for … (list as many things as you'd like)
- I deserve love and respect.
- I am valuable and contribute to the world around me.
- I am powerful and capable of success.
- I am manifesting _____ (what is needed for your goals?)
- I am powerful and capable of _____ (what is it you want to do?)
- I give thanks for _____ (the thing you want to do. See and feel it as if it has already happened.).

- I am living an extraordinary life in _____ (name of town where you want to be).

- I am blessed and abundant.

- I am limitless and free.

- I surround myself with positive people who encourage me to reach my goals.

- Wealth and abundance freely flow to me.

A highly effective way to absorb your intentions is to record them using your own voice. This is an easy way to program your subconscious mind as you only need to say them once while recording them. Then, all you do is listen during future therapy sessions. You can listen while you drive or when you are sleeping. Record at least 15 minutes of your intensions, even if you must repeat them over and over.

It is important that you use your voice to record your affirmations to make your subconscious mind more receptive to them. Ensure you feel positive and confident before you record your statements and intentions. Record all your statements in the same confident tone. Make sure that you believe everything you hear yourself saying. If the words cause resistance or tension in your body, go back to your written affirmations and rewrite them or choose words that you can say with integrity. Listening to your voice may feel uncomfortable initially, but rest assured, as you listen to your own voice, you will learn to empower yourself and trust in your own abilities. This practice is highly effective in so many ways. It helps to you become energetically aligned and worthy to receive. We must be proactive and set things in motion, taking action steps one by one to create what we want.

Laughter is the Best Medicine. We have all heard the saying laughter is the best medicine, and in fact, it has its own term: gelotology. Gelotology was established in the late 1960s by William F. Fry of Stanford University. It is the study of laughter and its effects on the body from both a psychological and physiological perspective.

Although laughter seems so simple, it is both complicated and subjective. It is a complex process, engaging multiple brain and body regions. The frontal lobe helps interpret the various bits of information received and decides whether something is funny. That triggers an emotional response in the limbic system, which controls feelings like pleasure and fear, which stimulate the motor cortex. We all love a good laugh, yet we rarely do it. Has it been far too long since you had a good, heartfelt laugh that lasted over 30 seconds—or where tears came to your eyes?

Studies show that laughing boosts the immune system by increasing immune cells and infection—fighting antibodies to improve disease resistance. It also lowers stress hormones, decreases pain, relaxes muscles, enhances oxygen intake, it improves digestion, and it prevents heart disease. Additionally, increases the antibody IgA (immunoglobulin A), which fights upper respiratory tract infections. And best of all, increases the number and activity level of natural killer cells that attack virally infected cells and some cancer and tumor cells. And let's face it—laughter raises our vibration.

Many movies and books claim that people have cured their illnesses through laughter. One of my favorites is the classic where Norman Cousins claims to have laughed his way back to health after his doctor gave him a few months to live after being diagnosed with a rare, crippling, and irreversible connective tissue disease. He was told to go home and get his affairs in order. The year was 1964. His stubborn and courageous nature wasn't buying this news. He fired his doctor, acquired a movie projector and a pile of funny movies including the Marx Brothers and Candid Camera shows and laughed his ass off, along with his new therapy of mass doses of vitamin C injections. His attitude, effective natural treatments, and laughter bought him 26 additional years! His experience was portrayed in his best-selling, groundbreaking classic, *Anatomy of an Illness*. He later died on November 30, 1990.

Laughing also enhances our emotions and nervous system by adding enthusiasm to life, improving mood, and releasing stress, anxiety, and fear. It is literally impossible to feel anxious, angry, sad, or scared when we're laughing. And it's contagious (in a good way)! Laughter works with the brain to reduce the level of stress hormones like cortisol, adrenaline, dopamine, and growth hormone. It also increases the feel-good hormones like endorphins, and neurotransmitters.

Laughter is fun, easy, spontaneous, and, best of all, it is free. Having this vital healing therapy at our disposal is convenient, but we have to remember to use it. Humor is subjective, and everyone will find different things funny. Watching something funny on TV, comedy skits, playing and sharing funny videos on YouTube, reading humorous books, telling jokes, and even being tickled will all provide excellent therapy.

Forced laughter is also making its way into the healing arts. Laughter yoga clubs are popping up all over the world. Some people like this form of therapy while others have difficulty laughing in such settings if they feel forced or self-conscious. How you make it happen doesn't matter. By making a conscious effort each day to at least have a chuckle or two will benefit your wellbeing. But let's shoot for that hardy laugh.

Words to Live By. Have you ever known someone, even for a very short time, who said something that stayed with you for the rest of your life because it profoundly impacted you? About twenty-six years ago, I worked as a paralegal at a law firm in Irvine, California. Within this law firm, a delightful woman named Linda worked as one of the firm's legal secretaries. She was a beautiful, heavyset Hispanic woman who was always cheerful and bright, and she made a hot salsa that, to this day, remains the best I have ever tasted. She was witty and had a way of making people laugh. I remember trying to persuade her to audition at comedy clubs.

At the time, there was a humorous diaper commercial that went something like this: *Johnny has a saggy diaper that leaks*. I later adopted that saying when I was having a bad day. One day at work, after an annoying situation, I was walking past Linda's cubicle and randomly stopped and said, "Linda, I have a saggy diaper that leaks." Without any hesitation, she said, *"then change it."* I was genuinely in awe of her prompt response—and of the simplicity and wisdom behind her valuable advice. All these years later, I barely remember anyone's name where I once worked, yet I remember everything about Linda and her profound words to live by.

If we choose to get out of the *saggy sagas*, we can. Whether it is the way we choose to view a particular situation or if circumstances are causing a situation to be intolerable, we have the power to change it. More than likely, the issue causing the diaper to leak in the first place will not even be remembered a week or month later. I have no idea what caused my distress that day. It wasn't important in the scheme of things. However, if it is a situation that is significant to the outcome of your safety or happiness, consider the following things:

- What about the situation is upsetting you?

- What would you need to do to improve the situation?

- What is stopping you from taking action today?

- If a lack of funds or other obstacles are standing in your way, what resources are out there for you to explore?

Being stuck in a situation that doesn't serve the soul will wreak havoc on the body, mind, and spirit. Being complacent or complaining about the situation is not a valid solution and does nothing to change it. Go within to discover ways that will inspire your inner spark to return. There is nothing you can't do if the desire is there. Take one step today to set it in motion. For example, talk to a career or life coach, travel agent, social worker, relocation specialist, etc. Embracing optimism is key to feeling hopeful and positive, and it can be a powerful catalyst for change. Feel the new energy circulating when you create optimistic scenarios and take action. But most importantly, if you have a saggy diaper that leaks, **change it!**

The Art of Acceptance. One of the biggest detriments to our happiness is resisting the present moment when things aren't going our way. Imagine getting into your car for an important meeting, and your car won't start. Do you automatically spin out of control, or take a deep breath and deal with what needs to be done? We can experience greater peace and fulfillment when we choose to practice acceptance. The art of acceptance is our journey to self-empowerment and contentment. It is not something we are born with. It is something we need to consciously practice daily. When events occur that are beyond our control, we have a choice to either learn the art of acceptance or make ourselves miserable as we struggle to change the unchangeable. Either way, the same result transpires whether it is handled with grace or in a stressful, frazzled, irrational way.

Acceptance is appreciating a moment or experience exactly as it is, without a label of *good* or *bad*. One of life's greatest lessons is learning to surrender and go with the flow. Life happens and it is our reaction and interpretation of the circumstances that will either free us or limit us. Once we stop fighting against "what is," we begin to notice the blessings that were always there. In the lessons inside the struggle, the beauty lies within the mess, the strength that hardship awakens. Acceptance clears the fog so that gratitude can see clearly.

Acceptance is being okay with any aspect of your life whether it is a particular situation or a life circumstance that you condemn. Trust that your life is unfolding perfectly in every moment. Forcing things to happen will create suffering, resistance, and struggle. Learning to trust in a higher power and letting go of the need for circumstances to be a certain way will liberate you and put you on the path toward self-mastery.

Oftentimes, we have a plan for our lives. Yet, often, our plans unravel for various reasons. Depending on our attachment to the plan, the outcome of any diversion from it may cause major upheaval and unhappiness. Being flexible to life's circumstances allows us the freedom to accept that something better than we could have imagined may be around the corner. The following poem from an unknown author sums it up quite nicely:

> When our plans unravel, threads of chaos weave a new tapestry. The fractured pieces, once disparate, now interlock in a dance of reconstruction. It's as if entropy itself conspires to birth something unexpected—a mosaic of resilience. In the shattered symphony, dissonance becomes harmony. The broken bridges lead to undiscovered shores, and the cracks in reality are hidden constellations. Amidst the falling debris, there lies a promise of renewal. So, when life crumbles, remember, chaos births creation, and sometimes, falling apart is merely falling into place.

It is important to remember that God's dream for our lives is so much bigger than our own and will take place in divine timing. If we were to receive an opportunity we wanted so badly (that we didn't receive) before we were ready, we might not have been prepared for the challenges, and failure may have prevailed. It's also possible that we thought we really wanted something that we may not have wanted at all. Learn to live wholly from the place of total acceptance and be willing to recognize challenges as lessons for self-growth. This is an important step on our sacred journey toward higher consciousness. Practice mindfulness and observe life without getting caught up in it or reacting to it. It is truly empowering. And always thank God for unanswered prayers.

And lastly (this is a tough one), it is important to accept the people in our lives just as they are—with unconditional love. So often, we try to change our spouse, children, friends, and family members if we don't approve of how they are orchestrating their lives or if they don't follow our beliefs. This is stressful for all parties involved. Remember, we are all living out our soul plan. If people want our advice and direction, they will ask. Our opinions and guidance are not to be force-fed to others. In fact, it will usually backfire and push them the opposite direction if they are not ready or willing to hear our opinions and suggestions. If you are truly concerned, you might consider beginning a topic with, *May I make a suggestion*? Always convey messages with love and respect, without judgment and attachment to the outcome; and, of course, with acceptance.

In response to each challenge that crosses your path, practice cultivating acceptance. Simply allow things to be without judgment and resistance and begin to notice the shift that begins to take place.

As the saying goes, *let go and let God*. And so it is . . .

Regaining Your Childlike Wonder. Let's face it: our adult lives have seemingly become too busy with too many chores, bills, debt, deadlines, responsibilities, and too much drama regarding family, work, relationships, finances, and politics. As adults, we often take ourselves too seriously, and in the process, we lose sight of ourselves and our zest for life.

Think about it. As an adult, when was the last time you skipped just for the hell of it, threw snowballs, made s'mores, cannonballed into a swimming pool, swung on a swing, rode on a merry-go-round, opened a wrapped present with enthusiasm, danced in the living room, sang like no one was listening, or looked at something in complete awe? When was the last time you had fun and felt like you were *being* a kid again? Granted, those with young toddlers are somewhat coerced into childlike activities and get a second chance to be a kid again. For those of you who are enjoying that period in your lives, are you fully engaged in it, or is it sometimes a chore? Are you on the phone or looking at your watch while walking with your dog or playing with your children?

As kids, we naturally had an innate curiosity and a lively determination to understand the world around us. We lived in a world where anything was possible, and adventure lurked around every corner. As toddlers, we were not yet aware of our peers or concerned about how others perceived us. We were without responsibility. We were barefoot and carefree. We were also naturally mindful.

We all have at least one friend who never acts their age or seems to be enjoying life a little more than they should. Are they wired differently? Are they considered to be immature? Do they perceive life differently than most people? Are they checked-out from reality? Well, it just happens that they've got it right. According to psychologists, all work and no play has serious consequences, both physically and mentally. When our inner psyche is repressed, we fail to reach our full potential. Something may feel wrong or off. We suffer from a sense of alienation, become restless, and feel a deep-seated sense of loss, leading to depression. Maintaining a sense of awe throughout life stimulates creativity. Albert Einstein attributed his sudden scientific breakthroughs to his childlike sense of wonder and curiosity. He was always asking himself why things were as they were, much to the annoyance of his teachers. Einstein sought to comprehend the inner workings of the universe, down to its most fundamental particles. His ambition to understand everything was immense. His life's goal was no less than to capture the beauty, the power, and the majesty of the universe into a single equation.

Why do we start to lose our sense of wonder in adulthood? Did our hearts become bruised and broken, or has the mundane juggling of our day-to-day chaos left our spirits too shattered to have a little fun? Are we too concerned or insecure about what someone would think if we did something goofy? The truth is, beneath all these layers of complication, we are all children at heart who are trapped and want to come out to play and connect with our surroundings. How can we reignite the spark in our lives?

The good news is that it is possible to rekindle our childlike awe and sense of wonder, even with all the punches life throws at us. It all starts with being mindful and present.

Spending time with fun-loving people will also bring fun moments. Laughing and being silly whenever possible is entertaining and often surprisingly contagious. Doing something out of your comfort zone can also create wonder, especially when doing it for the first time. What would you like to do or try that you have been putting off? Make a list and commit to doing at least one fun or new thing each month.

And lastly, allow yourself enough time to be present in all that you do. Always being in a hurry is a good way to miss out on what's going on around you, as it places the focus on where you should or need to be instead of where you are.

For further exploration and ideas on this topic, bestselling author John

O'Leary goes into depth in his book entitled, *In Awe: Rediscover Your Child-like Wonder to Unleash Inspiration, Meaning, and Joy.*

Speak Your Truth. Being truthful can create more happiness than you may realize. When we care about what others think of us, we often agree to things that we don't have time for or would rather not do just to gain approval. When we try to control what others think about us, it's like going through life with a bunch of masks and wearing the one that pleases the person in front of us to get their praise. Quite frankly, it is a burden—and a happiness killer!

When we are not being true to ourselves, we give our power away when we agree to do something or be someone we do not agree with. Such circumstances could be an employer asking you to do something that you are uncomfortable with, a parent who persuades you to marry a person you do not love, or coaxing you into choosing a college curriculum that may offer a higher salary than the one you would have preferred to study. It could be a friend asking you to lie about something. It could be a client demanding too much of your time, above and beyond the call of duty. The list can go on and on. Next time this happens, and you feel resistance, this is your opportunity to shine and simply *just say* "no". But say it with sincerity and love.

From this day forward, assess your choices and ensure that the decisions you make are in your best interest. Pay attention to your body and notice if feelings of dread arise when you are in a situation where you start to feel manipulated or controlled or if you begin to cave in and conform to someone else's expectations. If someone is creating a guilt trip for you by not complying with them or calling you selfish for not wanting to do something that doesn't work for you, notice if you are experiencing resentment, doubt, or resistance. Analyze the cause of these feelings. Be honest with yourself and others. Making the correct decision should feel good, not like a burden. If you feel any resistance, bow out with grace.

Communication guidelines to contemplate when corresponding what is truthful for you:

1. Am I responding out of fear or anger?

2. Am I responding out of obligation or guilt?

3. Am I dealing with this situation lovingly?

4. Is my solution based on the highest good for everyone involved?

5. But most importantly, use your words. And say them with love!

The Power of the Present Moment. If you blink, you may miss it! Why is being present so important? Because the present moment is all we have. The events of yesterday no longer exist, and tomorrow is an illusion. Yet, we usually find ourselves someplace other than where we are, thinking about something we did, need to do, or say next. How often do we find ourselves in a conversation contemplating our response and not being fully present to what the speaker is conveying?

Practicing presence gives us access to a powerful state of being that many people don't often utilize. In the famous words of Confucius, "*Wherever you go, go with all your heart*" he was encouraging presence and authenticity. When we go with all our heart, we're not just physically present. We are emotionally and spiritually invested in what we're doing. We act with alignment between our thoughts, feelings, and actions. This creates a deep sense of peace and joy, because our inner world and outer world are in harmony. In modern, holistic terms, it reminds us that energy follows intention. When we pour our full heart into life, our work, our relationships, our healing, and our purpose, we raise our vibration and invite more meaning into every experience. Going with all your heart isn't about perfection; it's about being fully alive in the moment you're in.

Setting an intention to be present when you leave the house, whether for an important meeting or a simple errand, allows for a more harmonious experience and a positive attitude. When we are truly in the present moment, it is impossible to experience worry, anxiety, or fear because these emotions are brought on by anticipating something that has not yet happened. Bringing our full attention to the present moment and what we are doing, opens a space that is free of random and habitual thoughts.

Starting with our beloved smartphones—look around the next time you're out and about. In restaurants, gyms, stores, and even out walking, nearly 80% of the people—from teens to seniors—have their heads buried in their cellphones with no awareness of what is happening around them. We are all guilty of this occasionally, but a beautiful world is passing us by. Sadly, we are all becoming more programmed and robotic without realizing it. We even text to communicate with friends and family, completely losing that human connection of hearing another person's voice. Making a conscious effort to break away from these chains that bind us can help us be present and notice our surroundings more vividly. Next time you are out doing a particular activity, put your phone on silent mode and try engaging with your senses. You deserve a break from your phone, even if it's just for one hour. The world can live without your cell presence for a short time. All that you may have missed will be there waiting for you next time you tune in.

Attachments and the Art of Letting Go. Much of our unhappiness arises from clinging—clinging to people, possessions, outcomes, identities, or old stories that no longer serve us. These attachments create invisible cords of expectation and fear: fear of loss, fear of change, and fear of being without what we've grown used to. When we hold on too tightly, we block the natural flow of life and keep ourselves stuck in emotional cycles that drain our joy. Unhealthy attachments often stem from the belief that something outside of us will complete or validate us. But true peace can never be found in things that are temporary; it comes from within—from the knowing that we are already whole.

Letting go doesn't mean we stop caring or disconnect from life—it means we release the need to control it. It's an act of trust, a surrender to the wisdom of the universe and the unfolding of our own path. To break free from unhealthy attachments, we begin by noticing where our energy feels heavy or dependent. We can practice gratitude for what was, forgiveness for what hurt, and acceptance for what is. Meditation, journaling, breathwork, and mindful awareness help us loosen our grip and return to center. When we let go with love, we create space for something greater to enter—freedom, peace, and a deeper, more authentic joy.

Letting go is not a single act. It is a process of softening, releasing, and trusting. It begins with awareness. Take a few quiet moments to breathe deeply and center yourself. Then ask:

What am I holding on to that no longer feels light?

Is this attachment helping me grow, or is it keeping me bound to fear, guilt, or expectation?

What would it feel like to set this down, even for a moment?

Visualize the attachment as an energy cord connecting you to the person, situation, or belief. With each breath, imagine gently loosening that cord—not cutting it in anger, but releasing it with love and gratitude for what it once taught you. You may even wish to affirm silently:

"I release what no longer serves me. I trust the flow of life and open my heart to peace."

End this practice by placing a hand over your heart, feeling the lightness of that space. Letting go creates room for joy, creativity, and new beginnings. It reminds us that freedom is not found in holding tighter—it's found in trusting that what is meant for us will remain, and what is not will gracefully fall away.

A Sense of Community: Natures Prescription for Happiness and Vitality. In an era of digital connection yet growing emotional disconnection, one of the simplest and most powerful determinants of health may be the people around us. The communities we belong to—our families, circles of friends, spiritual groups, and neighborhoods, play a profound role in our overall well-being. In fact, the science of longevity shows that community is not just comforting, it's life-extending.

We need to belong. People are wired for connection. From an evolutionary standpoint, our ancestors survived by banding together for safety, food, and shelter. That instinct to belong still runs deep in our biology. Modern research reveals that loneliness and social isolation are as harmful to health as smoking fifteen cigarettes a day. Chronic isolation increases inflammation, suppresses the immune system, and accelerates the progression of disease.

When we feel genuinely seen, supported, and accepted by others, the body relaxes. The parasympathetic nervous system—the body's "rest and repair" mode—activates. Heart rate slows, stress hormones drop, and oxytocin, the bonding hormone, rises. These physiological changes foster balance in our emotional and physical systems, from the brain to the gut to the immune response.

Being part of a community also gives life meaning. When we know that others rely on us, whether as parents, mentors, neighbors, or friends, we experience a sense of *ikigai*, a Japanese word for "reason to wake up in the morning." This sense of purpose is not abstract—it directly influences health. Studies show that individuals who identify a strong purpose in life have lower rates of heart disease, stroke, dementia, and depression. In moments of hardship, community provides resilience. Grief, illness, or financial stress become more bearable when shared. Mutual care transforms suffering into growth, reinforcing the truth that healing is often a collective process, not a solitary one.

Across the world, researchers studying the *Blue Zones*—the five regions with the highest concentrations of centenarians—discovered a striking pattern. Whether in Okinawa (Japan), Sardinia (Italy), Nicoya (Costa Rica), Ikaria (Greece), or Loma Linda (California), people live longer and happier not because of one miraculous diet or supplement but because they are deeply embedded in strong, supportive social networks.

In Okinawa, Japan, residents belong to *moais,* tight-knit groups of lifelong friends who meet regularly to share food, conversation, and mutual support. Their social bonds buffer stress and encourage healthy habits naturally. In Sardinia, Italy, multi-generational households are common, where elders remain respected and integrated in family life. Daily laughter, shared meals, and connection to village traditions keep their spirits and immune systems strong. In Nicoya, Costa Rica, community is central to the "plan de vida," a shared purpose rooted in faith, family, and helping others. This sense of belonging nurtures both the heart and mind. In Ikaria, Greece, neighbors drop by unannounced, share herbal teas, dance late into the night, and never eat alone. Their longevity is fueled by joy, connection, and a rhythm of life that honors human interaction. In Loma Linda, California, the Adventist community thrives on shared values of faith, plant-based eating, and service. Their spiritual and social cohesion protects against stress and chronic disease. In all of these regions, community is a way of life. People look after one another, and in doing so, they create an energetic field of love, purpose, and belonging that sustains vitality into advanced age.

From a vibrational perspective, community amplifies our frequency. When people gather with shared intention, their energy fields resonate, creating coherence—a phenomenon observed in studies of heart-rate synchronization and group meditation. Love, gratitude, laughter, and compassion elevate vibration not just individually, but collectively, uplifting the entire group. When we isolate, our frequency drops. We may feel disconnected, lethargic, or anxious. But when we engage by sharing meals, music, rituals, or even a simple conversation, the energy of community replenishes our soul. It reminds us that we are not separate; we are all one expression of a larger field of consciousness.

To experience these benefits, you don't need to live in a Blue Zone—you can create one where you are. Begin by nurturing authentic relationships built on trust, empathy, and shared values. Join a local wellness group, yoga class, or community garden. Host regular dinners or potlucks where everyone contributes. Volunteer for a cause that aligns with your heart. Reach out to friends you haven't spoken to in a while. Create rituals of connection such as morning walks, tea with neighbors, or family game nights.

True wellness extends beyond diet and exercise; it thrives in the soil of human connection. As we nourish our relationships, we nourish our vitality. When we give love freely and receive it openly, we participate in the same energetic harmony that sustains life in the Blue Zones—a reminder that health is not just a personal achievement but a shared one.

In fact, studies show that when people retire, that without the daily activities of work or the sense of belonging that comes from a shared purpose, many retirees begin to feel invisible. Studies show that this disconnection can take a serious toll on health when people lose their social ties after retirement of reporting a significantly higher risk of illness and even early death. Research has found that social isolation increases the risk of premature mortality by more than 30 percent, rivaling the dangers of smoking or obesity! When we lose our sense of purpose, identity, and connection to others, our biology takes notice. The body's stress hormones rise, inflammation increases, and the heart, both physically and emotionally, weakens. So, retirees, after the initial excitement of enjoying your newfound freedom of no work responsibilities, alarm clocks, or answering to anyone, wears off, it is important for vitality and longevity not to become complacent. Remember as new stages of life, maintaining community isn't simply a choice; it's a form of medicine. Join clubs, volunteer, start a hobby group, or simply share more meals with loved ones. A vibrant social life nourishes not only the spirit, but the cells themselves.

Chapter 25
Consciousness & Mindset

The Power of Consciousness. Within each of us lives pure awareness, a quiet observer, so to speak. Alongside it, is a louder companion referred to as the egoic mind. The ego was never meant to be the enemy; it was designed as a protector. Its purpose is survival. It scans for danger, plans ahead, and keeps us safe in a world filled with threats. However, those same protective instincts often keep us trapped in cycles of fear, worry, and self-limitation—if we let it.

The egoic mind thrives on identification; *"my job, my body, my story, my beliefs"*. It measures, compares, and defends because it believes that separation ensures safety. It whispers, *"Be careful. Don't trust. Don't fail. Don't stand out."* It keeps us replaying the past to avoid pain and projecting into the future to control the unknown. Its intention is good for wanting to keep us from harm, yet its methods often pull us away from the present moment, where peace and true power reside.

Fear is the ego's language. It tells us we are not enough, that we must do more, have more, and prove more. It thrives in busyness and distraction, because stillness threatens its control. The more we identify with the voice of the ego, the more we live in survival mode by reacting instead of creating and defending instead of trusting.

But beyond the egoic chatter lies our higher consciousness. This is the magnificent part of us that observes without judgment, that knows we are more than our thoughts or roles. This awareness allows us to witness the ego with compassion rather than resistance. When we begin to see the ego for what it is (a well-meaning but overactive guardian) we can thank it for its service and gently reclaim the driver's seat.

The journey of consciousness is not about destroying the ego but transcending its fear-based control. It's learning to listen with awareness instead of obedience and to let love, intuition, and truth become our new guides.

Consciousness is the essence of who we are—the awareness behind our thoughts, emotions, and actions. It is the silent observer that perceives life through us, shaping our reality in every moment. When we begin to understand that consciousness is not just the mind's activity but the awareness that holds it, we unlock the ability to consciously participate in the creation of our lives. Our state of consciousness determines how we experience the world, whether with fear or love, limitation or possibility, resistance or flow.

To shape our consciousness is to shape our health, happiness, and vitality. When our awareness expands, our perception changes, and so does our physiology. Science has shown that our thoughts and emotions directly influence our biochemistry, impacting hormones, immune response, and cellular communication. A mind anchored in gratitude, compassion, and optimism sends coherent signals to the body that promote healing and balance. Conversely, a consciousness clouded by fear, judgment, or negativity can trigger stress responses that deplete energy and vitality.

There is a distinct difference between being *conscious* and *unconscious*. Conscious living means acting with awareness and making choices that align with our highest values and well-being. Unconscious living, on the other hand, is reactive and automatic; it's when old patterns, limiting beliefs, and societal conditioning steer our behavior without reflection. Much of our suffering arises from this unconscious state—when we drift through life unaware of how our thoughts and emotions shape our reality.

Mindset is the bridge between consciousness and daily life. It's the lens through which we interpret our experiences. By cultivating a growth-oriented mindset, one that sees challenges as opportunities for expansion, we begin to live consciously. This practice transforms not only how we think, but how we feel, heal, and interact with the world.

Ultimately, elevating our consciousness is the highest form of healing. It's the realization that we are not victims of circumstance, but active participants in the unfolding of our destiny. When we awaken to that truth, health, happiness, and vitality become natural extensions of who we are.

The following sections explore different areas of consciousness and are meant for reflection and self-discovery. They offer opportunities to pause, look within, and consider how we might think, act, and perceive life in new, more empowering ways. Each area invites us to awaken a deeper awareness of ourselves and to recognize where subtle shifts in perspective can lead to greater peace and clarity.

Mindset is Everything. Mindset is the state of mind in which we organize and orient our thoughts and feelings about the world and ourself. Our beliefs hold the greatest power over the outcomes in our lives, both good and bad. A negative mindset impacts our ability to handle stressful situations because our negative thoughts will prevent us from coming up with solutions and keep us focused on the problem instead. Furthermore, a negative mindset can get in the way of our success, happiness, and our mental and physical health.

Generally speaking, a negative mindset is based off of limited beliefs such as, "I can't...," or even "I can try..." (which is a noncommittal attempt at doing something based on the fact that one may fail). When people are stagnant in their thought patterns, they cannot see outside of the reality they have created. Such beliefs such as *"I can't afford it. It's too risky. I don't have the time. I'll try. I could never accomplish that. I'll never find a good-paying job. I'll never lose this weight. Why don't good things ever happen to me? I'm incurable. That would never work. Rich people are not trustworthy. I'm not smart enough. I'll never get married."* etc. These thoughts create their reality because they believe it to be true. To change this reality, these thoughts need to be changed.

If you say you can't do something, it programs your subconscious mind to make it happen. For example, verbalizing things to yourself like, *I'll never learn that. I'm not good enough. I'll never get married. I'll never meet the right person. I'll never be happy. My life sucks.* Voila! It's like magic. Your words are your command! If one thinks they are a victim, then they are a victim. Just think about what you can accomplish with a positive mindset!

The good news is we can take action to reprogram our minds to focus on life more positively. You may be thinking, how is it possible in our world to be positive when there's so much negativity, fear, scarcity, violence, illness, and other annoyances thrown at us from every angle, from the television and newspapers to the collective consciousness. We don't need to feel guilty for not choosing to suffer because others suffer. It is crucial to cultivate a positive mindset and attitude so that we don't go down with the ship. We need to start accepting that our view of the world is a choice, and optimism is a learnable skill. Decide that the world is a positive place and that there is as much good as evil. Make the decision to release any resistance to this concept and accept it as your newfound truth, and try to ditch thoughts, feelings and beliefs that may be filling us with negativity.

When we live with low vibrational states of self-doubt, fear, and unworthiness, we stifle our ability to change, succeed, and thrive. We stay complacent in a reality that we no longer want. We get stuck in our limited reality due to our limited beliefs. The first step is becoming aware of the limiting beliefs we have about ourselves and how they impact our choices. We can do this through self-reflection. By doing this, we will become aware of how our mind has held us back. Being aware of our limiting patterns, we can stop them in their tracks and choose to believe something different. When we notice limiting thoughts & beliefs filling our minds, we can observe them and let them go rather than feeding into them.

A positive mindset is a perception that creates our reality and is open to everybody regardless of their circumstances. You, and you alone, are the only person you can change or have control over. Begin by noticing your inner dialogue. Throughout the day, pay attention to how often your thoughts lean toward worry, comparison, or judgment—of yourself or others. These are signs the unconscious mind is on autopilot, repeating old narratives that no longer serve you. Awareness itself begins to dissolve their power. When you notice a negative thought, *ask yourself, is it helpful? What would a more loving or empowering perspective be?"* This simple act of questioning interrupts the old pattern and invites the conscious mind to take the lead. Over time, this practice rewires the brain for optimism and resilience. Reframing challenges also helps. Instead of thinking, *"Why is this happening to me?"* try, *"What is this teaching me?"* A growth-oriented mindset turns obstacles into opportunities for expansion. Science supports this shift: positive thinking has been shown to strengthen immunity, reduce stress hormones, and improve longevity. Let's focus on some reflective questions:

- What negative thought patterns do I notice repeating most often? (For example: self-doubt, fear of failure, guilt, comparison, or scarcity.)

- Where do these thoughts originate? Are they my own beliefs, or have they been inherited from family, culture, or past experiences?

- How do I feel physically and emotionally when I entertain these thoughts? (Notice the energy shift in your body—tightness, heaviness, fatigue.)

- What is a more loving or empowering truth that could replace each negative belief?

- When I imagine living from this new mindset, how does my body feel? How does my energy change?

Our Perception of Reality

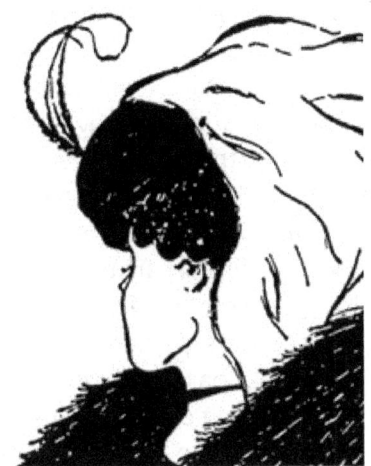

This famous photo has been circulated on the internet for years and has been studied and debated by psychoanalysts and philosophers numerous times regarding how the mind perceives things. Do you first see a young lady or an elderly woman? This illustration is a perfect example of the human mind and how we each interpret different perspectives regarding life's experiences. One can have a perception without being right or wrong because the mind creates our own perceived reality. In the example of this illustration, whether you saw a young lady or an older woman, you were right because they are both in the photo. So, does reality exist, or is our perception just an illusion? Is reality based on the electrical signals from our brain, which allow us to perceive what we see, smell, feel, and taste, or is it much more? And who decides what is *real*?

Our perception of reality is not an objective truth. It's a personal interpretation shaped by our thoughts, beliefs, emotions, memories, and sensory experiences. We share the planet with roughly eight billion people, all with different beliefs, perceptions, and realities that differ from our own. Two people can live through the same event yet perceive it in entirely different ways because each filters reality through their unique state of consciousness. The mind constantly interprets what it sees based on past experiences and internal narratives, often coloring the present with old patterns of fear, expectation, or desire. In essence, we don't see the world as it is, we see it as *we are*. By becoming aware of these filters, we can begin to shift perception from reaction to awareness, allowing us to see life through the clearer lens of truth, compassion, and higher consciousness.

There are basically two types of perceptions in how we interpret situations. For example, if you have a glass of water that is filled to the middle of the glass, one perspective would be that the glass as half full and the other perspective would be to see it as half empty. This phenomenon of perception can have a profound impact how we experience life. Those who view the glass more toward the glass-half-empty perspective, are said to have a negative perception. This type of perception affects all areas of our lives and spills over to relationships as well. For instance, people who perceive their spouse, boss, business partner, etc. as always being against them, they will most likely react in a defensive, reactive, and victim-like way, causing unease, unhappiness, paranoia, and negativity. This type of thought pattern is of a low, fear-based, vibrational energy that will draw the energy to attract what is being created in their mind. As you can see from this example, perception is subjective and creates our reality. Cognitive biases, emotions, past experiences, and cultural influences often shape our perceptions. By becoming more aware of how these factors influence us, we can align our view of the world more closely with objective reality. Most importantly, we must acknowledge that our happiness and fulfillment in life are our own responsibility and not that of others. Our circumstances do not determine our happiness; it is our interpretation of those circumstances and the meaning we attach to them that determines our happiness.

In conclusion, when we awaken to the truth that our outer world mirrors our inner state, we reclaim the power to create a more harmonious reality. Consciousness becomes the bridge between thought and experience, allowing us to shape our lives through awareness rather than reaction. As we lift our perception to a higher frequency—one of love, gratitude, and clarity—the world around us responds in kind. Life begins to flow with greater ease, synchronicities appear, and even challenges reveal deeper purpose. In the end, the more we expand our consciousness, the more radiant and whole our reality becomes.

Fear vs. Love. At the deepest level, all emotions stem from one of two sources: *love* or *fear*. Every feeling we experience—joy, peace, gratitude, and compassion—arises from love. Every emotion that causes contraction—anger, guilt, jealousy, shame, or anxiety—stems from fear. Love expands; fear constricts. Love heals. Fear separates. These two forces shape the vibration of our consciousness and the quality of our reality.

When we operate from love, our energy flows freely. We feel connected to others, open to life, and aligned with trust, harmony, and abundance. Our body responds with coherence, heart rate steadies, breathing deepens, and our cells communicate more efficiently. Conversely, when we live from fear, we disconnect from that natural flow. The body tenses, stress hormones rise, and we unconsciously move into protection rather than creation.

Recognizing which energy we are operating from in any given moment is one of the most powerful forms of self-awareness. Every thought, word, and action either expands us or contracts us. When we pause and ask, *"Am I choosing from love or from fear?"* we shift from reaction to consciousness. That single moment of awareness has the power to change our entire vibration—and with it, our health, relationships, and life experience.

Some examples of traits based on fear: Scammers—Poverty mindset based on fear of lack; Jealousy—Fear of losing love; Resentment—Fear of not having what others have (money, love, etc.); Possessive—Fear of loss of a person; Worry—Fear that something could happen; Insecurity—Fear of being judged; Bully—Fear of not being in control; Flamboyant—Fear of not being noticed; Disagreeable—Fear of other's beliefs—And on and on it goes...

One of the greatest acronyms of all time is:

FEAR – **F**alse **E**vidence **A**ppearing **R**eal.

Fear often feels real, but most of the time it's an illusion. The mind projects "what if" scenarios that rarely happen, yet the body reacts as though the threat is immediate. This is how the unconscious mind keeps us in survival mode, replaying old memories or imagined futures instead of allowing us to experience the calm and safety of the present moment.

When we pause and examine our fears, we often discover that the evidence behind them is anticipated, exaggerated, or imagined. Fear thrives on assumptions, not truth. By shining the light of awareness on it, we strip fear of its power. The moment we recognize that fear is often just a story the mind tells to protect us, we can choose a higher response of one rooted in faith, trust, and love. In that moment of clarity, fear transforms into wisdom. We realize that most limitations exist only in perception, and when we see through the illusion, our energy is freed to create, heal, and live fully.

The Media keeps us in fear as long as we allow it to do so. The news is designed to capture attention, and the easiest way to do that is through fear. Headlines are crafted to trigger emotional reactions (alarm, outrage, and worry) because fear keeps us watching. When we constantly expose ourselves to negative or sensationalized stories, the brain interprets this input as a real and immediate threat. The body then responds by activating the stress response, releasing cortisol and adrenaline as if the danger were happening to us personally.

Over time, this steady stream of fearful messaging trains the mind to look for what's wrong instead of what's right. It can create a subtle background anxiety that clouds judgment, weakens the immune system, and erodes our sense of safety and hope. We begin to see the world through a lens of danger and division rather than connection and possibility. Consequently, a recent client of mine was suffering from severe stomach pain and digestive issues. We were able to pinpoint the root which was her contempt and rage from the war scenes of children starving and hurt in her country of origin.

We must consciously choose what we allow into our awareness. Choose balanced, uplifting, or solution-oriented sources. Limit daily exposure and balance it with time in nature, meaningful connection, music, or meditation. The goal is not ignorance, but energetic protection by staying informed without becoming consumed. When we take charge of what enters our consciousness, we reclaim our peace, clarity, and trust in life's natural goodness. Awareness expands when fear no longer dictates what we see.

Advertising sells through fear. Much of modern advertising is built on the psychology of fear—specifically, the fear of not being enough. Marketers know that fear triggers a primal response in the brain. When we feel insecure, inadequate, or left out, we're more likely to buy something that promises to make us feel better, safer, younger, or more accepted. Advertising subtly plays on our deepest worries: *What if I don't look good enough? What if I miss out? What if I'm not successful, desirable, or safe?*

By presenting a problem (whether it's wrinkles, germs, debt, or loneliness) and then offering a product as the solution, advertisers tap into the subconscious mind, linking relief and happiness to consumption. These messages are repeated so often that they can become internalized as truth. Over time, we may begin to equate self-worth with appearance, possessions, or social status. This conditioning quietly undermines confidence and fosters a cycle of striving for more instead of feeling content and whole. Yet awareness is liberation. When we cultivate self-mastery, we can see through the illusion, and even smile, knowing our value has never depended on anything external.

Becoming conscious of these tactics is liberating. When we see how fear-based marketing works, we can step back and ask, *"Do I truly need this, or have I been taught to believe I do?"* Conscious consumers make choices from empowerment, not insecurity. When we buy or support something from a place of alignment, because it enhances health, joy, or authenticity, we shift from fear-driven consumption to love-driven creation.

Along those lines, there is a difference between how we view being a disciplined eater and a mindful eater. A disciplined eater may make certain dietary decisions based on the fearful belief that eating certain foods may cause them harm, such as fatigue, disease, or weight gain. Alternatively, a mindful eater will make dietary choices to keep their body healthy, fit, and balanced. While both may be making the same healthy choices, can you feel how they are coming from different places energetically?

As our consciousness grows, we can see through the illusion of fear. Fear loses its grip the moment we bring it into the light of awareness. Most fears live in the imagination, projected into the future or replayed from the past. Rarely do they exist in the *present* moment. When we return to the here and now, the mind quiets, the body relaxes, and we remember that, in this moment, we are safe.

Find a comfortable space, take a deep breath, and place your hand over your heart. Feel your breath move in and out steady and effortless and ask yourself:

- What fear has been taking up space in my mind lately?
- Is this fear based on something happening *now*, or is it a projection of what *might* happen?
- What is the actual truth of this present moment?
- If I were to respond with trust instead of fear, what would that look like?
- What small step could I take right now that aligns with peace, not panic?

As you breathe, imagine your fear as a cloud gently dissolving in the light of awareness. Each exhale releases its hold, bringing you back into the calm, grounded energy of the present. When we live in the present moment, fear cannot survive, because it feeds on uncertainty, not truth. Presence reminds us that right now, all is well, and from this place of peace, clarity and courage naturally arise.

Transcending Duality. Humanity has long viewed the world through the lens of duality—light and dark, good and bad, right and wrong, us and them. This way of perceiving reality creates contrast, which is necessary for learning and growth, but it also fosters division when we forget that both sides exist within the same whole. Transcending duality means rising above polarized thinking to see life from a higher perspective, one that embraces unity, balance, and understanding.

From birth, we are conditioned to categorize the world around us. We learn what's acceptable and what's not, who belongs and who doesn't, what's "right" versus "wrong." These early perceptions shape our sense of identity and reality. Yet these are *learned perceptions*, not absolute truths. What one culture praises, another may reject. What one person fears, another may cherish. When we realize that every belief is filtered through experience and conditioning, we open the door to empathy and humility.

Duality isn't inherently bad. It's part of the human experience. Without contrast, we wouldn't recognize beauty, joy, or light. Can you imagine how boring a football game would be if the entire stadium were rooting for the same team? It's when we cling too tightly to one side of any spectrum, we fall into judgment, conflict, separation, and in some dire circumstances, hatred and violence. Transcending duality asks us to expand our consciousness by holding multiple truths at once and to understand that opposites often serve the same divine purpose: awakening to greater awareness.

True consciousness honors diversity. Every soul's journey is unique, shaped by personal lessons, backgrounds, and karmic paths. What someone believes today may be exactly what they need for their own evolution—and that truth may look very different from ours. Our truths can also change and be completely different a day, a month, or a year from now.

When we encounter opinions that challenge us, the ego wants to defend and prove itself "right." The heart, however, seeks understanding. By choosing curiosity over judgment, we soften the barriers between each other. This doesn't mean agreeing with everything. It simply means respecting the right of others to see through their own lens. Wisdom is not found in convincing others to think like us, but in holding compassion for those who don't.

In a world increasingly divided by ideology, politics, and belief systems, transcending duality is more important than ever. Division keeps humanity in a lower vibration—one ruled by fear, anger, and resistance. Unity consciousness, by contrast, operates through love, acceptance, and connection.

Transcending duality doesn't mean erasing differences; it means recognizing that beneath all differences, there is an underlying oneness. Just as day and night are both necessary for the rhythm of life, so too are the varied perspectives that make up humanity's collective growth. When we look beyond labels and opinions, we see that every person is an expression of the same source energy.

When we release the need to label life as good or bad, success or failure, we begin to live in a more fluid and peaceful state of being. Every situation becomes an opportunity for growth. Instead of asking, "Who's right?" we begin to ask, "What can I learn here?" Instead of reacting to opposites, we integrate them.

This higher awareness frees us from emotional turbulence and reactivity.

We begin to see life as a dance of energies, where all contrasts serve our evolution. In that space, we no longer fight reality—we flow with it.

Our conscious path forward to transcend duality is to live from the heart rather than the ego. It's to recognize the divine in all things—even in the people or experiences that challenge us most. As consciousness expands, judgment fades, replaced by compassion and understanding and observing without labeling, and listening without defending. In this elevated state, we see not a world of opposites, but a field of harmony—a universe perfectly designed to awaken our soul to its own radiant truth.

Reflect and Integrate: Transcending duality begins not with changing others, but with observing ourselves. It's about catching ourselves when we want to judge, divide, or label (and we will!), and choosing instead to feel compassion. Find a quiet space, take a few deep breaths, and let your awareness settle into your heart. Reflect on the following questions to bring more balance, openness, and compassion into your consciousness:

- Where in my life do I tend to see things as strictly right or wrong, good or bad?

- What happens to my energy when I feel the need to defend my beliefs or prove a point?

- Can I honor another person's truth without needing it to match my own?

- What lessons might my "opposite" or "trigger" be here to teach me?

- How would my perspective shift if I saw everyone, including myself, as doing the best they can from their current level of awareness?

Mindfulness and Practicing Presence. Simply stated, presence is about being fully aware and engaged in the current moment, free from distractions and mental clutter. This allows us to connect with our thoughts, feelings, and surroundings, fostering a sense of peace and clarity. It allows us to enjoy the *now* moment as opposed to sleeping though it. When our heads are not buried in our cell phones or in deep mental clutter, we may have a chance to see and feel the world around us. Perhaps it's opening or holding a door open for someone walking into a store at the same time you are, allowing a person with one item in a checkout line to go in front of you when you have a full cart, starting a conversation with a stranger, petting a dog or engaging with a baby, smiling at a stranger for no reason at all, or simply looking up at the bright blue sky, realizing what a beautiful day it is. These are the moments where we can shine our light and make a difference.

Why is being present so important? Because the present moment is all we have. The events of yesterday no longer exist and tomorrow is an illusion. Yet, we usually find ourselves someplace other than where we are, thinking about something we did, need to do, or say. How often do we find ourselves in a conversation already contemplating our response and not being fully present to what the speaker is conveying?

Practicing presence gives us access to a powerful state of being that many people don't often utilize. Setting an intention to be present when you leave the house, whether for an important meeting or a simple errand, allows for a more harmonious experience and a positive attitude. When we are truly in the present moment, it is impossible to experience worry, anxiety, and fear because these emotions are brought on by anticipating something that has not yet happened. Bringing our full attention to the present moment and what we are doing, opens a space that is free of random and habitual thoughts.

Starting with our beloved smartphones, look around the next time you're out and about. In restaurants, gyms, stores, and even out walking, nearly 80% of people—from teens to seniors—have their heads buried in their cell phones with no awareness of what is happening around them. We are all guilty of this occasionally, but a beautiful world is passing us by. Sadly, we are becoming more programmed and robotic without realizing it. We even text to communicate with friends and family, completely losing that human connection of hearing another person's voice. Making a conscious effort to break away from these chains that bind us can help us become more present and notice our surroundings with greater vividness.

Being mindful is of particular importance when cooking and eating. Practice mindful cooking when preparing meals. What is your mood? Are you stressed? Angry? Are you multitasking as you are focusing on a chaotic situation? It is important to be mindful of your thoughts and emotions while touching and preparing food because negative energy can be transferred into meals and absorbed by the recipients. Before chopping, dicing or slicing anything, express gratitude for the meal you are about to prepare and for each ingredient you are working with. Smell and appreciate the aromas of the seasonings and herbs. Realize the healing benefits of each nourishing ingredients being used. Take your time. Feel the texture of each item as you chop. Treat each move as a meditation. Be creative. Play inspiring music. Cook with love. These practices raise the vibrational frequency within the foods you will be eating.

Mindful eating is a beneficial practice that can be easy to forget, especially when we're on the go. It is a practice that involves being fully present and engaged during the act of eating. It is good practice for both our physical and emotional health. Begin by giving gratitude before any meal. It is just as effective whether you prefer to do it out loud in the form of a prayer or internally with your thoughts. Give thanks for the nutrition you will be receiving. Give thanks for the vegetables that grew for you. If you are eating meat or seafood, give thanks and show deep gratitude for the sacrifice that was provided to nourish our bodies. Be mindful of each bite by chewing slowly. Savor the flavors. By eating slowly and chewing thoroughly, we will have better digestion and absorption of nutrients.

Always eat in a healthy environment. Never argue or debate with anyone during a meal. If you enjoy watching television while eating, avoid watching the news or shows that promote violence or contain contentious material; as these energies can negatively impact your digestion. Keep it light and enjoyable. Better yet, play soothing music and eat by candlelight. Enjoy the outdoors, when possible, and eat alfresco. Being mindful of how much food you eat is a great practice. Not being present while eating can easily lead to overeating. It is always a good idea to stop eating when you feel just slightly full, then remove the plate from the table.

Get Grounded! We've all heard the term "getting grounded" but what does it really mean, and why is it important? Imagine a large oak tree deeply planted into the earth, with its roots stretching over six feet deep. It is well grounded in the soil and can withstand any disturbances that may come along with ease. Other trees with more shallow root systems may tumble over in stormy weather. Much like a tree, we also need to have a firm foundation to anchor ourselves to Earth, mentally, physically, and spiritually. When we're not grounded, we're like a leaf in the wind, light and easily vulnerable, and highly reactive to adverse situations.

When we feel like life is throwing us a curveball and situations become more stressful than we would like, it is easy to be thrown off balance. Doing some simple grounding exercises can help bring awareness back into our center to be more mindful. It allows us to weather the storm much easier so we can withstand these challenges with more balance and peace. Grounding is also a basic core daily spiritual practice within personal development to help us feel connected energetically to the earth's core. Scientifically speaking, grounding has positive health benefits such as the power to reduce inflammation, enhance immunity, improve sleep, reduce cortisol levels, relieve pain, and calm the sympathetic nervous system (great for stress!).

The easiest grounding technique we can do is called *earthing*. We can automatically connect with the earth's energies by standing or walking barefoot on the ground or grass. For those fortunate enough to have a beach nearby, my number one recommended healing remedy is walking barefoot on the shoreline. Take deep breaths in and out and visualize your feet taking root into the earth's surface. By grounding, we are absorbing the earth's electrons—called negative ions—which neutralize our charge and balance our bodies at the cellular level. Negative ions can also be experienced around moving water such as streams and waterfalls, mountain terrains, and even after a thunderstorm.

Grounding or earthing mats mimic this connection by providing an electrical link between our body and the earth. The idea is to replicate the physical connectivity one would make by walking barefoot on the ground. These devices can certainly be helpful; however, I will always prefer nature over electricity whenever possible.

Another way to obtain life-force energy is from a deeply rooted tree. Trees radiate natural healing energy that can help restore balance and vitality. When you find a tree you feel drawn to, it's proper to ask for permission with a simple, "May I?" Its grounding capabilities can transfer to all who seek them. After you have absorbed its energy, remember to thank it. One word of caution from experience: make sure your tree is free from ants or other critters before working with it!

Spending time in nature, hiking and gardening are also great ways to connect with the earth and relieve tension.

Using Your Words Effectively. Our words are powerful and hold vibrational energy—they can heal or harm, uplift or diminish, inspire growth or sow doubt. Every word we speak carries a vibration that ripples through our environment, shaping not only how others feel but also how reality unfolds around us. Spoken with love and intention, words can spark hope, nurture confidence, and open hearts. They have the ability to transform energy, bridge divides, and plant seeds of change that can blossom into extraordinary outcomes. When we choose our words consciously — with kindness, truth, and compassion — we become alchemists of light, using language as a force for healing, connection, and transformation.

No doubt, confrontation is not fun for the average person. For some, however, it can almost seem like a hobby. The art of effective communication is to set aside one's ego and convey the message with love. For example, how many times have you or someone you know had a complaint about a bill or service issue and handled it by angrily yelling at the customer service representative? The service rep is getting their head bashed in while the company is being maligned. The communicator's adrenaline and blood pressure climb sky-high. I once had a situation where I was on the receiving end of such a call. I asked the customer, "How can I fix this situation for you?" There was a long pause. They were so focused on being angry that they didn't have a solution to resolve their issue.

When people communicate any message with a higher state of consciousness, the tone will be calm and concise, and they would have asked for a fair solution. The receiver of the message would be far more willing to help a rational, pleasant person than a nasty one. How many times have you had a boss, spouse, parent, friend, or even a stranger approach you in uncivilized communication? How did you react? Would you have responded more favorably if they had communicated the same message with different words or softer tones? Alternatively, have you flown off the handle for something that you could have conveyed more effectively? How would you do it differently today?

On the flip side, a lack of communication is when we have a problem, complaint, or criticism about someone and choose not to confront the issue. This is one of the worst things we can do to ourselves as this negative energy will build up in the form of hurt, anger, resentment, and regret. It may not be apparent at the time, but it will explode in other ways in the future and will always occupy a space in our minds until it gets resolved—no matter how small or large the issue may be.

Many years ago, my best friend and maid of honor—unbeknownst to me—had a grudge against me. Her way of handling it was to cut off our communication without any explanation. Sixteen years later, she contacted me after listening to a forgiveness CD her business partner shared with her, discussing what had happened and how she had interpreted the situation. Because of this misunderstanding and lack of communication, we lost sixteen years of friendship, and I missed participating in her child's life as he grew up. A simple conversation would have cleared it up immediately.

And lastly, we should look at the relationship we have with words in our daily lives. We are all guilty of using unfavorable words from time to time. Whether we use them on ourselves, our children, friends, spouses, or others, now is the time to clean up our language. How many times a day can we catch ourselves spewing out toxic words? Examples are, *you idiot, stupid, messed up* (or explicitly, *f'd up*), *I hate, I can't, I'm so fat,* etc. Let's start transmuting those words the moment they arise—and start spreading love, even to ourselves.

Gratitude: The Frequency That Changes Everything. Energetically speaking, everything in the universe operates through frequency and resonance. When we live in a state of appreciation, our vibration rises, aligning us with the frequencies of abundance, love, and joy. According to the Law of Resonance (which underlies the Law of Attraction), like attracts like. When you consistently broadcast gratitude, you magnetize experiences, people, and opportunities that match that high vibration.

Gratitude is more than a fleeting emotion. It is a state of mind, a way of seeing the world through the lens of abundance rather than lack. It's the awareness that life itself is a gift, and that even the simplest moments, a bright blue sky, a quiet moment, walking with a friend, are blessings waiting to be noticed.

Gratitude is also a choice that we make every day. We may not control what unfolds around us, but we can always choose how we respond. Even in hardship, gratitude invites us to find meaning to look beyond what's missing and honor what remains. This choice doesn't ignore pain; it transforms it. It softens the heart, calms the mind, and brings coherence back into the body.

Science now confirms what ancient wisdom long knew: when we practice gratitude, we activate regions of the brain that cultivate joy, empathy, and emotional balance. The nervous system relaxes. Stress hormones drop. The body shifts out of survival and into harmony. Gratitude, quite literally, changes our chemistry. In fact, it is physically impossible to be stressed and grateful at the same time.

Gratitude grows when we shift our perception by choosing to see the same situation through a higher lens. It's not about forcing positivity; it's about recognizing the quiet blessings that already exist within everyday life shown by these examples:

Instead of saying, *I have to pay these bills,"* think to *yourself, I get to pay these bills — because I have a home, electricity, and running water."*

Instead of thinking, *I'm exhausted from work,"* try, *I'm grateful for meaningful work that supports my life and gives me purpose."*

Instead of complaining, *"I have so many chores,"* reframe it *to, "I get to care for my space — a reflection of the life I'm blessed to live."*

Even moments of discomfort can be invitations for acceptance and gratitude:
"This challenge is teaching me resilience."
"This delay is guiding me toward divine timing."
"This ending is creating space for something new."

The practice of noticing, reflecting, and shifting is simple yet profound. When we choose gratitude in the small things, life expands in beauty and meaning. We begin to see that every breath, every sunrise, every interaction holds a gift waiting to be acknowledged. It is not reserved for the perfect days; it is what makes ordinary days feel extraordinary.

Give Consciousness a Spin with FLFE!

They say that money can't buy happiness—but just maybe it can buy consciousness! Imagine, just having to enter your physical address in an on-line database, and receive a high consciousness energy field in your home or place of business. Focused Life-Force Energy (FLFE) is a consciousness technology that focuses and activates a high consciousness field that produces results very similar to a person praying for a person or place. The FLFE System redirects and focuses Life Force Energy (also known as Chi, Prana, and Mana), which is present throughout the universe. The purpose of the system is to activate a consistently positive environment for us to thrive. The service supports us in creating a nurturing environment to expand our consciousness, rest more deeply, boost our body's natural innate healing, increase our mental function, and energize our environments.

FLFE is a field of consciousness with calibrated statements, which they call programs. It's like automated affirmations or prayers that are calibrated to 999 or higher on the Hawkins Map of consciousness. It would be like having thousands of monks praying for your well-being, your health, your family, and your property, 24/7.

The way that this is accomplished is via a machine; imagine something a bit futuristic and related to Nikola Tesla's work. The machine is made of stacks and contains many different things such as precious metals, crystal spheres, and sacred geometry. This machine draws in and focuses life-force energy, which is connected to our database of property addresses and phone numbers. The energy within the machine communicates through this universal field to activate the FLFE bubble around your home or phone.

I have been a subscriber for nearly seven years. You can log in and change your address anytime you move or go on vacation, so the energy is always there surrounding you and your family. It's definitely worth logging onto their website to read what it's all about and learn about the inventors and research. This phenomenal technology currently has over 13,000 Subscribers in over 86 Countries. And for fun, you can experience it completely free. Focused Life-Force Energy offers free trials for both property and mobile service for 15 days (no credit card needed for the trial). https://www.flfe.net.

Chapter 26
Emotional Healing Through Self-Reflection

Self-reflection is consciousness in motion. It is both *awareness of being* and the *practice of presence*. Cultivating it benefits mind, body, and spirit, helping us live with more peace, clarity, and authenticity. Self-reflection, shadow work, and soul diving allow us to explore our inner terrain where unprocessed emotions, limiting beliefs, and old wounds quietly shape our choices and well-being. When practiced with compassion and nonjudgement, we reprogram our psyche with the wonders of who we truly are and discard beliefs that no longer serve us.

Self-reflection. Simply stated, self-reflection is the intentional practice of pausing to look inward, examining your thoughts, emotions, beliefs, and behaviors to gain insight into yourself. It can be done through journaling, quiet contemplation, meditation, or simply setting aside time to review your day or week. Unlike casual daydreaming, self-reflection is purposeful: you are observing your inner life to understand motives, identify patterns, and align with your deeper values. Through reflection, we are not dwelling or rehashing something that would be easier to brush under a rug forever. Instead, we are bringing it to the surface and into the light to heal and let it go.

This simplified example demonstrates how Maya's story unfolded and how these healing journeys begin:

It was late evening when Maya finally closed her laptop, hoping her assignment would please her demanding boss. The house was quiet, but her mind raced with unfinished conversations and a vague heaviness she couldn't identify. Instead of numbing her thoughts with television, she sat on her living room floor with her journal. At first, only scattered thoughts came. Then, as she kept writing, an old memory surfaced—her father's sharp words when she was eight. Tears followed, but so did a calm clarity: the tension she'd been feeling at work wasn't about her boss; it was an unhealed wound she had carried for decades. That night marked the start of her journey inward.

Self-reflection is just that. There are no set of rules for a successful practice. It is more of a personal preference on where and how you would like to do it as well as the length of time you would like to invest. Journaling about a challenging conversation and what you learned from it as well as writing about daily events, emotions, or key questions like "What am I grateful for today?", taking some quiet moments in meditation to simply notice thoughts, emotions, and sensations without judgment, going on contemplative meditative walks alone, spending a few minutes each night asking what went well, what could improve, and how you felt., start a blog reflecting on your experiences to engage others who may be dealing with similar issues, or simply chatting with a counselor, friend, or spouse about your thoughts.

Self-reflection has helped numerous people to realize unresolved trauma that keeps the nervous system on high alert—a state that can compromise immunity, digestion, and mood, identify triggers that caused sudden flares of anger or sadness brought on by a word or sound, and suppressed negative emotions that can surface as chronic headaches, fatigue and cause dis-ease in organs correlating to specific organs. Also, when working with self-sabotaging patterns like procrastination, perfectionism, or unhealthy coping habits, we can often trace them back to unmet needs or unhealed stories. Further, our repressed emotional state can distort our view on how we perceive things which can negatively affect our relationships, mood, stress, happiness, and wellbeing by keeping us in victim mentality. When we meet these parts of ourselves with compassion, the energy once bound in pain becomes available for creativity, vitality, and authentic connection.

Shadow Work: The Force Behind What Makes Us Tick. I like to describe shadow work as self-reflection on steroids. Shadow work is like digging a little deeper into our psyche to identify, integrate, and heal the parts of ourselves that usually stay hidden from the light of day. These "shadows" are the emotions, traits, and impulses we suppress or deny—anger we don't want to admit to, jealousy we pretend isn't there, trapped emotional energy, memories, fears, or emotions we've repressed because they feel shameful or painful. Left unacknowledged, the shadow can quietly influence our thoughts, reactions, and even our health.

The Swiss psychiatrist Carl Gustav Jung first coined the term *shadow* to describe these unconscious aspects of the psyche. He taught that true wholeness comes not from perfection but from embracing all parts of the self, light and dark alike. When we engage in shadow work, we consciously invite those hidden aspects into awareness. In doing so, we restore lost energy, raise our frequency, and move closer to soul-integration, where every part of us resonates in harmony.

Before we go any further, if this work feels too uncomfortable, too *out there*, or too touchy-feely, that is perfectly fine. Emotional healing can be sought out when you are ready. It is not easy or fun. It requires discipline and the desire to face unpleasant memories, traumas and situations that are stored in our cellular memory. Just know that you are not alone. Not a single person on this planet is exempt from negative emotions, past traumas, childhood imprints, self-sabotaging patterns, and emotional blocks. If they have not been properly processed, they are stored in the conscious mind, subconscious mind, and passed down from one generation to the next through family lineage. They can even be emotions that you are holding for another person. If you take nothing else from this chapter, please understand that transformation is not about changing who you are—it's about discarding who you are not.

Soul Searching and Soul Diving: What Drives My Happiness?

Soul searching is an inner exercise of deep reflection where you turn inward to explore your true self, values, desires, and purpose. It's less about finding answers in the external world and more about uncovering the wisdom and guidance already within you. People often turn to soul searching when they feel lost, unfulfilled, or at a crossroads in life. Often, the terms *soul* and *spirit* are used interchangeably. However, I interpret them differently although they are deeply connected. The *spirit*, which is pure consciousness, is the life force energy within us—the breath of existence that animates the body and connects us to the divine. The *soul*, on the other hand, is our inner self, the seat of the mind, emotions, free will, and personal identity which also co-creates with spirit. When we live out of alignment with our soul's truth or intended path, inner restlessness arises, which can weigh heavily on the body and soul. This misalignment often manifests as emotional pain, stress, or even illness within the body. Here are some basic questions in this category to reflect upon:

Discovering Your True Self

- 1) When do I feel most authentically *me*?
- 2) What beliefs about myself have I outgrown, and which ones still hold me back?
- 3) What would I pursue if I wasn't afraid of judgment or failure?
- **Values & Purpose**
- 4) What are the three values I want my life to reflect the most?
- 5) If I had one year left to live, how would I spend it?
- 6) What legacy or impact do I want to leave behind?
- **Healing & Growth**
- 7) What wounds from the past am I still carrying, and what do they need in order to heal?
- 8) Which emotions do I avoid facing, and why?
- 9) What recurring patterns show up in my relationships or choices?
- **Alignment & Direction**
- 10) What in my current life feels aligned with my soul—and what feels out of alignment?
- 11) What drains my energy the most, and what restores it?
- 12) Which small steps could I take today to live more in tune with my deeper purpose?
- **Connection & Spirituality**
- 13) What practices make me feel most connected to something greater than myself?
- 14) Where do I feel the presence of peace, love, or spirit in my daily life?

- 15) How do I define a "meaningful life" for myself—not by society's standards, but my own?

Soul diving, on the other hand, is considered a deeper, more immersive practice of going *into* the soul's depths, often confronting hidden patterns, wounds, or unconscious beliefs to focus on healing, transformation, and integration of the shadow and subconscious aspects. It is a deeper, more intense dive – like plunging into the ocean rather than walking along the shore. It is less about "finding direction" and more about *revealing and integrating what's buried*, so you emerge lighter and more whole.

- Find a quiet, safe place to reflect and meditate on the following questions. Some may find it more beneficial to work on one at a time or cycle through several.

- 1) What do I most want to create in my life, if fear were not a factor?

- 2) What parts of me feel hidden, judged, or unexpressed?

- 3) What are the beliefs I hold about myself that I formed when I was young—do they still serve me?

- 4) When have I felt most alive, most aligned, or most "in flow"? What was happening then?

- 5) Which relationships or situations frequently trigger me—and why? What do these triggers reveal about unmet needs or unhealed parts?

- 6) If I could speak to my future self (5-10 years from now), what advice, wisdom, or warnings might they share?

- 7) What would it take for me to live more fully in my values—every day, not just on special occasions?

- 8) What parts of me have I neglected or repressed, because I didn't think they were acceptable or important?

- 9) What would I do differently if I truly believed I am worthy / enough / capable?

- 10) What are my deepest fears around love, success, or failure—and how might I be constructing stories around them?

Tools for Going Deeper. Often, when we discuss identifying subconscious blocks and emotions that hold us back, the first thing that comes to mind is: *How can I retrieve suppressed emotions if they're subconscious?* Just know that gradually, they will surface—one by one—once you start paying attention. Journaling and keeping track of triggers that appear, or noticing if a sudden feeling of resistance pops up and tracing it to its roots, can be extremely revealing. However, there are additional tools to help the emotional-healing process along more quickly. Some are specifically designed to identify blocks, while others are more basic self-reflection tools to get the juices flowing.

- **The Emotion Code** is an energy healing method developed by Dr. Bradley Nelson. Its core idea is that unresolved emotional experiences can leave behind "trapped emotions"—energetic residues of feelings like fear, anger, grief, or rejection—that remain lodged in the body long after the event has passed. According to this perspective, these trapped emotions may distort the body's energy field, contributing to physical discomfort, emotional imbalance, or even limiting beliefs and self-sabotaging patterns. The system was designed to identify and release these trapped emotions so that the body and mind can return to a more natural state of balance and harmony. Practitioners often use muscle testing (a form of applied kinesiology) to access the subconscious mind, identify which emotions are stuck, and then release them energetically, often with the help of intention and a simple magnetic technique. For more information visit: www.DiscoverHealing.com. If you are interested in working with an Emotion Code healer in your area, visit www.AlternativesforHealing.com.

- **SoulScans** a transformational emotional-well-being tool that detects hidden emotional and spiritual blocks, energetic imbalances, childhood imprints, self-sabotaging patterns, and negative emotions using remote (surrogate) bioenergetic testing worldwide. It comes with a do-it-yourself instruction manual for self-reflection and instructions for clearing. It also includes personalized affirmations. For more information visit: www.SoulScans.com.

- **Human Design** is a personal profiling system created in 1987 by Ra Uru Hu (born Robert Allan Krakower). It blends together several traditions and sciences, including Western astrology (based on your birth time, date, and place), The I Ching (Chinese Book of Changes with its 64 hexagrams), The Kabbalistic Tree of Life, The Hindu chakra system, Modern genetics and quantum physics concepts. Using your birth information, Human Design generates a chart called a BodyGraph. This map shows your energy centers (similar to chakras), how they are defined or undefined, and the way your personal energy flows and interacts with the world. A free personalized report is offered at www.Human.Design.

- **The Gene Keys** is a modern spiritual system created by Richard Rudd. It combines insights from the I Ching, astrology, the human genome, and contemplative practices to explore human consciousness and personal transformation. Each Gene Key represents a spectrum of consciousness with three levels: Shadow (unconscious patterns or challenges), Gift (awakened qualities when the Shadow is transformed), and Siddhi (the highest expression of that quality, representing enlightenment or divine realization). Designed to unlock higher potential by transforming limiting patterns into creative strengths and live with more compassion and authenticity by cultivating gentleness, forgiveness, and higher states of consciousness. By contemplating these Gene Keys, individuals gain insight into their patterns, gifts, and life purpose. Visit www.GeneKeys.com to receive your free profile.

Chapter 27
Meditation: The Science of Stillness

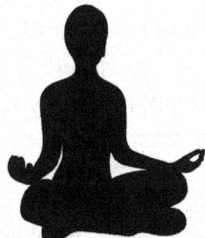

"Quiet the mind and the soul will speak." -Ma Jaya Sati Bhagavati

In our fast-moving world, stillness has become a rare treasure. Most of us spend our days rushing from one thought or task to the next, our attention constantly pulled toward screens, lists, and deadlines. The mind rarely gets a true moment of rest. Yet ancient traditions—and now modern science—agree on one truth: when the mind grows quiet, the body begins to heal.

Meditation isn't about stopping your thoughts or escaping reality; it's about training your awareness—learning to notice what's happening within you and resting in the present moment. Once practiced only in monasteries, meditation now fills the pages of medical journals, and the findings are nothing short of extraordinary.

Meditation is an excellent way to calm the nervous system. Stress is one of the greatest disruptors of health. When we live in constant "fight or flight," our bodies flood with cortisol and adrenaline, driving up blood pressure, weakening immunity, and accelerating aging. Meditation helps reverse this stress response.

A large review from Johns Hopkins University found that regular meditation eased anxiety, depression, and pain as effectively as certain medications (without the side effects). Harvard researchers discovered that after just eight weeks of mindfulness practice, activity in the brain's fear center (the amygdala) decreased while areas linked to emotional balance grew stronger.

Meditation has the ability to sharpen focus and mental clarity. Because our attention is constantly under siege by phones, notifications, and multitasking, the modern mind is overstimulated and fragmented. Meditation acts like strength training for the brain—building the "focus muscles" that help us stay centered and clear. Even ten minutes a day can make a measurable difference. Studies show improved memory, concentration, and problem-solving with consistent practice. Brain scans reveal why: meditation strengthens the prefrontal cortex (focus and decision-making) while quieting the "default mode network," the part of the brain tied to rumination and self-criticism. Whenever you feel foggy or forgetful, a few mindful breaths may be the most natural brain boost available.

Meditation doesn't just soothe the mind—it transforms the body. Research shows it can lower blood pressure, improve heart rate variability, and reduce pain and inflammation, one of the core drivers of chronic disease. The American Heart Association even recommends meditation as a complement to conventional care. By activating the parasympathetic nervous system (the body's natural "rest and digest" mode) meditation slows the heart rate, calms the nerves, and restores internal balance.

And last but not least, a peaceful mind may actually keep the body younger. Scientists studying cellular aging have found that meditation helps preserve our telomeres, the protective caps on our DNA that shorten as we age. Regular meditators have been shown to maintain longer telomeres and higher levels of telomerase, the enzyme that repairs them. In essence, meditation not only makes you feel younger, but it may also keep your cells younger, too.

The nice thing about meditation is that it is simple and free. It's not required to sit in a formal lotus body posture with our hands upward in the jnana mudra position, trek up the Himalayas, or attend an expensive spiritual retreat to get the most out of our meditation practice. In fact. it can be done sitting in a chair, lying on the floor, or walking in nature.

For those who are just beginning their practice, go small. For example, set an intention for five minutes. I like complete silence but some days

I prefer relaxing spa music (instrumental only) as background noise. Set your timer for five minutes. Take three slow breaths in and out and then breathe normally. If you wish, you could start with a few affirmations or close your eyes and ask, *what would you like me to know*? Then simply sit in silence for five minutes. Go into your practice with no expectations. When you find your mind wandering, go back to your breath and try to clear your mind. One trick that works when your mind is racing is to ask yourself, *I wonder what my next thought will be* and see what happens. Try to increase the amount of time each day until you reach at least fifteen minutes or longer as your schedule permits.

If sitting in silence is not the thing for you right now, brainwave entrainment in the form of binaural beats, can be an effective way for many people to get into a meditative state. This interesting phenomenon was discovered in 1839 by the German physicist Heinrich Wilhelm Dove. He found auditory beats form inside the brain when each ear is presented with its own tone of a slightly different pitch, allowing the electric rhythms of your brain to begin harmonizing with the same rhythms of an external source, causing hemispheric synchronization within the brain. As a result, we will experience a shift in consciousness and can access heightened levels of focus, creativity, relaxation, or even super-learning capabilities depending on the chosen beats. For meditation, theta-hertz frequencies play an essential role in getting us into that relaxation mode of our brain where emotional healing, intuition, daydreaming, and spiritual wisdom take place. People who use binaural beats claim to drop into that state quickly. Binaural beats are also known to have relaxing hypnotic effects. Headphones are required with this technique. You can find binaural beats online through different sources including YouTube. "Theta Waves Meditation" is a very good one.

PART THREE: BIOFREQUENCY FOR VIBRANT HEALTH

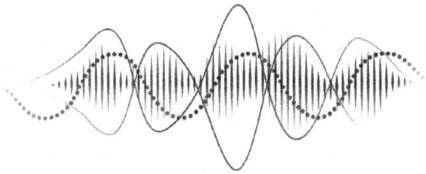

The Science and Spirit of Biofrequency Healing

Imagine if your body could "tune itself" the way a musician tunes an instrument—adjusting its inner frequencies until everything hums in harmony again. Every cell, organ, and thought vibrates at a specific frequency that reflects our state of health. When those frequencies fall out of balance due to stress, toxins, or emotional overload our vitality fades. Yet when we restore harmony through the intelligent use of frequency, the body remembers how to heal.

In this section, we explore the fascinating world of biofrequency and energy medicine—where modern technology meets the body's innate intelligence. We will discuss innovative tools that harness subtle energy to rebalance and recharge the human system. They don't override the body; they remind it how to return to coherence.

As you'll discover, frequency isn't just science—it's a language. A vibration that speaks directly to your cells, your nervous system, and even your emotions. When we learn to work with that energy, we open the door to deeper healing, expanded vitality, and radiant health from the inside out.

Though often labeled "alternative," these energy-based modalities are gaining ground in mainstream medicine. Their approach aligns with a growing recognition that the body is not just biochemistry—it's bioelectric and vibrational as well. In fact, even major medical institutions are beginning to integrate frequency therapies. A friend of mine who was being treated at the Mayo Clinic for a rare blood cancer, was recently prescribed red-light therapy as part of his recovery—a powerful sign that the tide is turning.

Today, thousands of energy-based healing systems exist—from clinical-grade modalities to at-home biofield devices. Some are FDA-cleared for specific conditions; others remain on the frontier of holistic practice. You'll find them offered by naturopathic doctors, chiropractors, wellness centers, and independent healers worldwide. As technology and consciousness evolves side by side, the boundary between science and energy medicine continues to blur—and the possibilities for self-healing expand with it. Throughout this section, we will discuss a handful of established therapies that have provided remarkable outcomes for both my clients and me. As time goes on, I expect to see many more innovative and beneficial ways to effectively promote healing with energy.

Chapter 28
Bioenergetic Testing

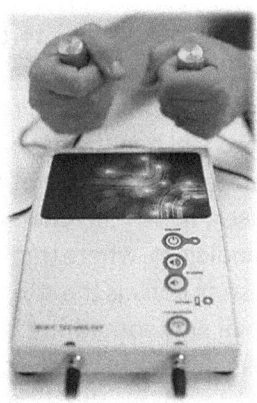

Bioenergetic Testing

What would you think if I told you there was a machine that can read your energy and tap into the inner workings of every cell in your body to discover the root cause of nearly every symptom, imbalance, and ailment to learn exactly what the body needs to heal? It requires no blood tests. It requires no invasive testing procedures, and you can get your results instantly. Better yet, that this invaluable tool can give insights as to why mysterious symptoms are occurring when conventional lab testing could not. It can also prescribe the exact remedy needed to put your body back into balance. And it's fast, painless, accurate, and affordable.

Too good to be true? Skeptical? **So was I!**

Twenty plus years ago, I was suffering from digestive issues. I did some research and decided to treat myself to a very expensive blood test to reveal what my food sensitivities were. I did a little more research and found a natural medical doctor in my area that advertised the exact blood test I wanted. He had an excellent reputation with many 5-star reviews.

On the day of my appointment, after chatting for a bit, he places me in a room where a practitioner greeted me with this exact machine (above). I immediately corrected him, explaining that I was there for the blood test. He waved his hand dismissively and said, *"This is way better."* I was taken back by his disregard for my request but decided to proceed with the appointment. To my surprise, the experience left me both skeptical and deeply intrigued. Despite not understanding how this "crazy machine" worked, I couldn't deny how incredibly comprehensive and insightful the health information it provided was.

Years later, when I decided to start a holistic wellness practice, I remembered the strange machine I once tried years earlier and ordered one for my practice. After all, it didn't make sense to tell people to eat spinach and other "healthy" foods if they were actually sensitive to them. For twelve years, this has been my primary go-to resource to help my clients determine what they need to feel healthy again. I have never had a client who wasn't completely amazed by this type of testing or the information they received. In many cases, it was life-changing. It's the perfect complement to conventional medicine—where traditional lab tests expose the symptoms, bioenergetic testing reveals the story beneath them. And when we discover the root cause of why something is not functioning properly, it can be addressed, treated, and often resolved rather than merely managed with medication that suppresses the symptoms.

How this Technology Began

In the late 1940s, Dr. Reinhard Voll—a German medical doctor and engineer—began researching and developing an innovative energetic testing procedure known as Electroacupuncture According to Voll (EAV). After more than a decade of hospital studies, this method became both documented and validated in Germany.

In the United States, EAV has continued to grow in acceptance, particularly among medical practitioners specializing in alternative and integrative medicine. Many professionals now consider it to be a significant advancement in the future of diagnostics and energy-based healthcare.

What is Bioenergetic Testing?

Bioenergetic testing is a computerized screening system that combines biofeedback, electrodermal screening, and meridian stress analysis all in one. It is used by hundreds of naturopathic doctors, cancer clinics, holistic health practitioners and wellness centers throughout the world to reveal functional disturbances on the cellular level. It is a non-invasive, state-of-the-art, quantum system that can either be done in person or remotely anywhere in the world for determining the root cause of imbalances within the body within minutes, simply by holding two probes while the tests are running.

At my center, we use the Qest4 (formerly called Asyra) for our screenings. After extensive research, I believe it to be the #1 bioenergetic testing system in the world due to its comprehensive capabilities and advanced software algorithms. However, there are many other manufacturers, and I will be the first to say that they are all remarkable tools as the information they provide is truly invaluable. The software contains digitally encoded information relating to a wide range of health factors that is output by the hardware as electromagnetic signals during testing. Using a simple low voltage circuit created by holding two brass cylinders or hand masses, the response of the body to those signals is recorded by measuring changes in the electrical resistance of the skin. This information is relayed back to the software, and a report is generated on the computer of any responses that are outside certain limits.

The system is used for testing imbalances within the systems, glands and organs. We can energetically identify immune disfunction, hormonal imbalances, neurological issues, gut and digestive imbalances, allergies, pathogens, Lyme bacteria, viruses, parasites, and fungi—as well as imbalances contributing to sleep disturbances, memory issues, ADD/ADHD, brain fog, depression, anxiety, and much more. It's important for patients to understand that these types of testing are not diagnostic. In other words, it will never tell you that a disease is present. The testing procedure delivers a picture of health status and how to correct it. Clients leave with a clear plan how to improve their health after just one visit.

How Bioenergetic Testing Works

In the purest form of bio-energetic testing, we are effectively asking the body a question and obtaining the response directly from the body's own physiology, without engaging the conscious and language centers of the mind. Although bioenergetic testing works through energy, every organ, gland, and system in the body—beyond its physical and chemical make-up—also holds an unseen energetic essence, a subtle field of information known as the energetic system. The subject of energy is an interesting subject and a bit overwhelming for many to get their arms around. In a nutshell, we are all energy. People (even animals and objects for that matter) have an energetic IP address, much like a cell phone or a computer. Our holographic nature allows these advanced devices to read our energetic field with incredible accuracy. It is helpful to make some comparisons to other similar techniques. Many people will be familiar with muscle testing or kinesiology, which is another form of bioenergetic testing applied by health practitioners. In kinesiology the question is often asked verbally, or the subject may hold an object or substance that is being tested. The response is measured by changes in the contractile strength of the skeletal muscles, checked manually by the tester. I often refer to bioenergetic testing as electronic kinesiology that measure the body's response to signal outputs from the device by recording and analyzing resulting changes in the electrical resistance of the skin.

Another informative comparison is the phenomenon of ideo-motor response, which is used by hypnotherapists. When a subject is in a trance state, a set of pre-defined response patterns (e.g. raising one finger or another, which occurs without conscious effort) can be observed to obtain responses to questions about which the subject may have no conscious recollection. This method can be used to recover memories from the unconscious mind, which is thought to store all our experiences, regardless of whether we can 'remember' them in normal consciousness.

These examples bear similarities to testing with our system however our testing goes one step further. The challenges or questions are presented by a micro-power radio signal output, rather than in words. The quantum nature of energetic testing devices has the capacity to broadcast healing frequencies to people and pets (such as homeopathics, herbs, hormones, emotional remedies, etc.) whether in the same room or across the world!

Through the science of quantum mechanics—a mysterious yet fundamental field that studies the composition of matter and how it behaves and interacts at the submicroscopic level—we have successfully performed thousands of remote scans with clients worldwide using just one piece of DNA from the client (saliva, a hair sample, fingernail clipping, or even a photograph) through the use of our surrogate technology. Remote screenings are just as effective as sitting in the actual screening room—although perhaps not quite as much fun.

Where to Get Tested

If you are interested in trying this type of health screening, simply do an internet search for "bioenergetic testing in [your city]" or "bioresonance or bioenergetic testing near me." As mentioned earlier, these scans can also be done remotely. However, if you have never experienced one before or are new to this type of procedure, I highly recommend scheduling your first session in person at a clinic. This allows you to see the process firsthand, understand how it works, and ask any questions that arise.

Bioenergetic Systems for Home Use

If you have an aptitude for technology and have ongoing health issues, larger families, or just desire optimal health, there are some very good and affordable options available to everyone. There is a bit of a learning curve but once you get through it, these technologies will be invaluable to you and your family—potentially saving thousands in healthcare costs over time. Personally, I cannot recommend one system over another, as I have not personally used them. However, many of my clients who own these devices have shared outstanding experiences and results. Both systems listed below offer informative videos on their websites that explain how each one works.

- **The Healy Device** (www.healy.shop). This popular handheld device delivers targeted healing frequencies at your fingertips and has earned high client satisfaction. Currently available in over 50 countries, it has been used in hundreds of thousands of applications and is supported by a growing library of positive testimonials.

- **The Genius Insight** (https://geniusinsight.app). This mobile application works with both Apple and Android devices and offers a comprehensive body scan using your voice signature and a selfie upload. Healing frequencies and balancing remedies can then be transmitted directly through the app. They also offer a two-week free trial period for new users.

Chapter 29
Rife Machines

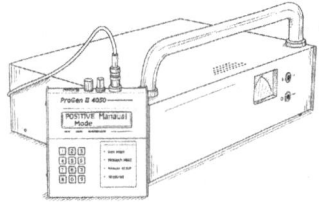

The Tainted History of Rife Technology: The Good, The Bad & The Ugly. There has been a lot of history, controversy, and speculation behind Rife frequency generators. This particular modality seems it can be singled out as an unaccepted technology by the Western medical system. More than likely due to the unthinkable claims of curing disease, namely cancer.

Theoretically, let's just hypothesize that if an inventor came along with any type of medical therapy not just to treat, but the possibility to *cure* cancer, wouldn't that be celebrated by every man, woman and child on the planet? Or would the large medical conglomerates want to condemn it and squash it to keep pharma intact? Afterall if there were cures for anything, the multi trillion-dollar medical industry, wouldn't be needed, and their treatments would become obsolete. According to the American Medical Association, the United States' health spending is projected to reach $5.6 trillion through 2025 and growing. Numbers hurt my head. I'm not a mathematician or a financial analyst, but in my humble opinion, this model simply doesn't align with cures.

American scientist Royal Raymond Rife, believed bacteria or viruses inside tumors emitted specific electromagnetic frequencies. He developed a high-powered microscope he claimed could detect these frequencies from bacteria and viruses by the color of their auras. In the 1930s, he developed another machine called the Rife Frequency Generator. He claimed it produced low-energy radio waves with the same frequency as cancer-causing microbes. He believed sending this frequency to the body would make cancer-causing microbes shatter and die. His work was built on the work of Dr. Albert Abrams. Abrams believed every disease has its own electromagnetic frequency. He suggested doctors could kill diseased or cancerous cells by sending an electrical impulse identical to the cell's unique electromagnetic frequency. This theory is sometimes called radionics.

The American Medical Association (AMA) and other medical authorities refuted claims of Rife technology, stating it was primarily due to the lack of scientific validation and evidence supporting Rife's theories, condemning his experiments, emphasizing the need for rigorous scientific validation and peer-reviewed research to support such claims. The Food and Drug Administration (FDA) never approved his inventions. To this day, Rife machines are not FDA approved for any type of illness or medical disease. Yet, even with the so-called best health care systems in the world and the best scientific advancements, heart disease and cancer are still the prevalent causes of death today even with the use of chemotherapy as the FDA approved drug for cancer treatment. It is unclear if there is an on-going vendetta between the powers that be and the manufacturers of frequency generators or what constitutes testing and the amount needed to prove an item worthy of approval. Afterall, the FDA has recently had over 14,000 drug recalls in the U.S., averaging nearly four recalls a day over safety concerns! One has to wonder what constituted rigorous scientific testing and scientific validation for the products that were originally approved to later learn they were (potentially) causing harm to the public?

As the story goes, an obituary in the Daily Californian described his death at the age of 83 on August 5, 1971, stating that he died penniless and embittered by the failure of his devices to garner scientific acceptance. Rife blamed the scientific rejection of his claims on a conspiracy involving the American Medical Association (AMA), the Department of Public Health, and other elements of "organized medicine", which had "brainwashed and intimidated" his colleagues.

Interest in Rife's claims was revived in some alternative medical circles by the 1987 book by Barry Lynes, *The Cancer Cure That Worked: 50 Years of Suppression,* which claimed that Rife had succeeded in curing cancer.

After this book's publication, various devices bearing Rife's name were marketed as cures for diverse diseases such as cancer and AIDS. Some used radio waves as in the original experiments, and some used other methods, such as pulsed electric current or pulsed electromagnetic fields at the correct frequencies or what the manufacturers believed to be the correct frequencies.

Rife devices were marketed with grandiose claims which led to health fraud warnings. In a 1996 case, the marketers of a Rife device claiming to cure numerous diseases, including cancer and AIDS, and removal of numerous pathogens were convicted of felony health fraud. The sentencing judge described them as "targeting the most vulnerable people, including those suffering from terminal disease" and providing false hope. Several arrests followed in subsequent years by health providers making outrageous claims in order to secure a healthy business.

Rife Machines Today. Rife frequencies are a hot topic in holistic health circles. As more people explore non-invasive, energy-based healing methods, this once-obscure technology is seeing a major revival. Rife frequency generators are highly regarded as excellent wellness tools to assist with the many health challenges of our toxic world. Although they are still not FDA approved, they are available for sale in the United States due to the fact they are classified as non-medical devices and can only be marketed as a wellness tool for personal experimental purposes. No claims should be made by manufacturers or practitioners as to any types of cures.

Rife Frequencies Explained. Just as the concept that pharmaceuticals are designed to have a frequency that matches the disease they treat (a process achieved through pharmacokinetics and pharmacodynamics), Rife frequencies also target specific Rife frequencies through specific electromagnetic hertz frequencies theorized to match the resonant frequencies of harmful pathogens. Everything that exists resonates with a certain vibration. As long as the mortal oscillatory rate (MOR) of the pathogen matches the frequencies of the resonance of the cause of the health issue, the organism will literally be shaken until the outer membrane breaks apart (much like when a singer can shatter a glass if a particular tone is reached).

According to the original theory, when these frequencies are applied to the body, they may disrupt or destroy viruses, bacteria, parasites, and other invaders without harming healthy tissue. While sitting in front of the machine, the frequencies are delivered through a plasma ray tube and delivered to the body. The trick here is to obtain the *exact* frequency needed for a specific issue. For example, if a patient has some type of food poisoning and they run a frequency for salmonella when it may be an E. coli infection, the frequencies used will not match the disease, and the patient's health won't improve. One way to make sure you have the correct frequency for the ailment is to get a firm diagnostic test from your doctor. Alternatively, you can check with your bioenergetic testing device. I understand that some Rife machines for home use, such as the Spooky 2, tests to identify the exact frequency needed.

Health Benefits of Frequency Generators. Although Rife frequency generators do not have the ability to cure any disease or ailment (see how I did that?), they can greatly enhance the cellular health of both people and pets. The ability to speed up the body's ability to heal itself has been witnessed firsthand. I have heard several testimonials from clients and healers who had debilitating illnesses (such as Lyme disease) that could not be helped through conventional means that attribute their health successes through the use of frequency generators. Today, machines are far more advanced than they were back in the day. They not only have the ability to eliminate pathogens but also perform thousands of tasks such as cellular regeneration, immune system support, detoxification, anti-aging, inflammation, circulation, emotional health, cognitive issues, and numerous wellness protocols. It's as simple as keying in the preprogrammed set number or hertz (if known), sitting back, and absorbing the healing frequencies. It can be used while sleeping, working at your desk, or watching TV.

How to Obtain a Rife Machine for Home Use. Rife machines vary in price from low-end models ($800), mid-tier models ($2K-$4K) and professional use models (4K-8K). My clients that use a Spooky2 love the device while others say there's a bit of a learning curve. Other reputable brands to check out for their ease and simplicity are the GB4000, Spooky2 Plasma, TrueRife, Beam Ray, and Resonant Light.

The Hulda Clark Zapper, while more limited in technology than Rife devices, operates using simple square-wave frequencies between 15 Hz and 500 kHz. It is claimed to help destroy pathogens such as bacteria, parasites, and viruses by disrupting their cellular membranes. Versions of the device are still available for purchase today.

Chapter 30
Acupuncture

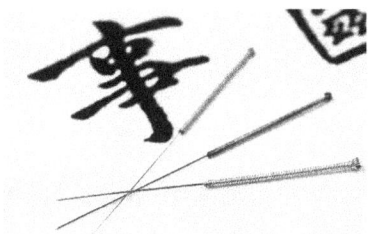

Acupuncture: Balancing the Body's Energy Pathways. Acupuncture is one of the oldest healing practices in the world, with origins tracing back over 2,500 years in China. Rooted in Traditional Chinese Medicine (TCM), it's built on the idea that the body's life force—known as Qi (pronounced "chee")—flows through a network of energy pathways called meridians. When this energy moves freely, health flourishes. When it becomes blocked or imbalanced, physical, emotional, or mental symptoms appear.

Acupuncture aims to restore harmony by stimulating precise points along these meridians, helping Qi flow smoothly once again. Today, acupuncture is recognized by both holistic practitioners and modern medicine for its ability to activate the body's natural healing mechanisms.

What the Procedure Looks Like. A typical acupuncture session begins with a consultation. The practitioner asks about your symptoms, energy levels, emotions, digestion, and sleep patterns, because in TCM, every aspect of your life offers clues about your internal balance. After your assessment, the practitioner selects a series of acupuncture points. You'll then lie comfortably on a treatment table. The practitioner gently inserts very thin, sterile needles (often no thicker than a human hair) into specific points on the body. Most people feel little to no pain, describing the sensation as a light tingling, warmth, or gentle heaviness. Once inserted, the needles are typically left in place for 20 to 30 minutes while you rest.

During this time, many people enter a deeply relaxed state. Some even drift into what acupuncturists call an "acu-nap", a state between wakefulness and sleep where the body's energy begins to recalibrate.

How Acupuncture Works: Ancient Wisdom Meets Modern Science. From the TCM perspective, acupuncture works by balancing the flow of Qi through the meridians, harmonizing the body's internal environment. But modern science has begun to uncover physiological explanations that align with these ancient concepts:

Nervous System Regulation:
Acupuncture stimulates sensory nerves under the skin and in the muscles. This sends signals to the spinal cord and brain, triggering the release of endorphins, serotonin, and dopamine—chemicals that reduce pain and elevate mood.

Inflammation Reduction:
Studies show acupuncture can decrease pro-inflammatory markers like cytokines and promote anti-inflammatory pathways, aiding healing in chronic conditions such as arthritis and autoimmune disorders.

Circulatory Support:
It enhances blood flow and oxygenation to targeted tissues, which accelerates recovery and nourishes organs.

Autonomic Balance:
Acupuncture helps shift the body from "fight-or-flight" (sympathetic mode) into "rest-and-digest" (parasympathetic mode), promoting deep relaxation and stress relief.

Although acupuncture is not technically a biofrequency modality, it clearly belongs in the broader energy and vibrational healing category. Each needle acts like a tuning fork, influencing the body's subtle energetic fields and creating measurable shifts in vibrational harmony. By restoring energetic coherence within the meridians, acupuncture helps recalibrate the body's electromagnetic balance—often producing profound emotional, physical, and even spiritual effects. In this way, it aligns seamlessly with other vibrational therapies that emphasize frequency, flow, and resonance as keys to wellness.

Medical Conditions Acupuncture Can Help With. Acupuncture's versatility is one reason it's become a cornerstone of integrative medicine. The World Health Organization (WHO) and National Institutes of Health (NIH) have recognized its effectiveness for a wide range of conditions, including:

Pain Relief: Back pain, neck pain, arthritis, sciatica, migraines, and fibromyalgia.

Stress & Mental Health: Anxiety, depression, insomnia, PTSD, and emotional imbalance.

Digestive Issues: IBS, bloating, nausea, acid reflux, and appetite regulation.

Hormonal & Reproductive Health: PMS, menopause, infertility, and low libido.

Immune Support: Allergies, asthma, autoimmune conditions, and fatigue.

Neurological Disorders: Headaches, neuropathy, Bell's palsy, and post-stroke recovery.

Addiction & Detox: Smoking cessation, alcohol withdrawal, and support during detox programs.

Many patients report not only physical improvements but also a greater sense of **calm, clarity, and emotional balance**—a testament to the holistic nature of the therapy.

The Healing Experience. A full course of acupuncture usually involves several sessions over weeks or months, depending on the condition. While some people feel results immediately, others notice gradual improvement as the body's energy recalibrates.

Because acupuncture treats root causes rather than just symptoms, it offers deep and lasting transformation. Regular sessions can enhance vitality, improve sleep, balance hormones, and support overall wellness—making it a powerful ally in a holistic lifestyle.

Acupuncture for Anti-Aging and Preventive Wellness. Beyond treating pain or illness, acupuncture has earned growing attention for its anti-aging and rejuvenating benefits, both physically and energetically. In Traditional Chinese Medicine, aging is viewed as the gradual decline of Qi, blood, and organ vitality. When these systems become depleted or stagnated, visible signs such as wrinkles, dull skin, fatigue, and slower metabolism begin to appear. Acupuncture helps revitalize the body's internal energy flow, stimulating regeneration from the inside out.

Facial acupuncture, sometimes called cosmetic acupuncture or acupuncture facelift, involves the gentle insertion of fine needles into specific points on the face and neck. This process increases circulation and collagen production, tones facial muscles, and encourages lymphatic drainage—resulting in a more radiant, lifted, and youthful appearance. The skin receives more oxygen and nutrients, giving it a natural glow without the use of chemicals or fillers. Many patients notice improved skin tone, reduced puffiness, softened lines, and a renewed sense of vitality that extends far beyond the surface.

Energetically, acupuncture also balances hormonal and adrenal function, enhances sleep quality, and increases overall energy flow throughout the meridians, contributing to a feeling of vibrancy and well-being that naturally reflects in one's complexion and demeanor. In this sense, beauty becomes an outward expression of internal harmony.

From a preventive health perspective, acupuncture is not only therapeutic but a great maintenance tool. Instead of waiting for symptoms to appear, many people schedule monthly or seasonal sessions to keep their Qi flowing smoothly and their immune and nervous systems in balance. This proactive approach supports emotional equilibrium, strengthens resilience against stress, and helps the body adapt more gracefully to life's changes.

In modern terms, acupuncture can be thought of as "energetic tune-ups" to fine-tune the body's internal frequency so that wellness, beauty, and vitality remain your natural baseline rather than something to chase after illness sets in. Regular maintenance acupuncture has been linked with better circulation, improved sleep, hormonal stability, mental clarity, and increased energy—all of which contribute to longevity and radiant health.

Chapter 31
Cold Laser Therapy

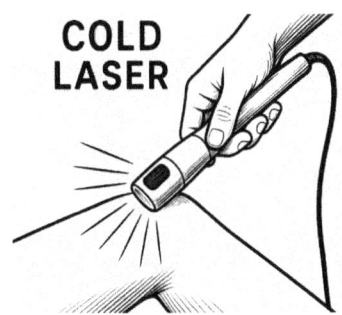

Cold Laser Therapy: Light as a Healing Force

In the ever-expanding field of energy and frequency medicine, cold laser therapy, also known as Low-Level Laser Therapy (LLLT) or photobiomodulation, stands out as one of the most scientifically validated ways to use light for healing. Unlike surgical or "hot" lasers that cut or cauterize tissue, cold lasers emit gentle, low-intensity light designed to *stimulate* rather than destroy. These subtle beams of red and near-infrared light penetrate below the skin's surface, triggering biological processes that enhance cellular repair, reduce inflammation, and accelerate healing—all without pain or heat.

Origins and Evolution

The story of cold laser therapy begins in the 1960s with Hungarian physician Dr. Endre Mester, who was researching the effects of laser light on cancer cells. To his surprise, instead of damaging tissue, the low-level laser he used caused the shaved backs of his experimental mice to grow hair more quickly and wounds to heal faster. This accidental discovery marked the birth of a new field called laser biostimulation.

Over the following decades, researchers in Europe, Russia, and later North America expanded on Mester's work, studying how light of specific wavelengths and intensities could influence biological tissues. NASA became interested in the technology in the 1990s to speed up wound healing and tissue repair in astronauts, a setting where the body's recovery mechanisms are challenged by microgravity. From these early studies emerged the modern concept of photobiomodulation, a term that better captures how light *modulates* cellular activity.

How It Works

Cold laser therapy operates on the principle that cells absorb photons, just as plants absorb sunlight for photosynthesis. When specific wavelengths of light—typically between 600 and 1000 nanometers—are absorbed by chromophores within the mitochondria (the cell's energy centers), they increase the production of adenosine triphosphate (ATP), the molecule that fuels nearly every biological function.

This boost in cellular energy can:

- Accelerate tissue repair and collagen synthesis
- Enhance circulation and lymphatic drainage
- Reduce oxidative stress and inflammation
- Decrease pain signals by affecting nerve conduction
- Improve mitochondrial function and overall cell vitality

Essentially, cold laser therapy helps the body return to energetic balance by *awakening dormant healing mechanisms* already present within each cell.

Clinical and Wellness Applications

Today, cold laser therapy is widely used in medicine, physical therapy, sports rehabilitation, veterinary care, and holistic wellness. Its versatility is remarkable:

- **Pain Relief & Inflammation:** For arthritis, tendonitis, bursitis, fibromyalgia, and joint pain. It reduces prostaglandin production and promotes endorphin release.

- **Wound Healing:** Speeds recovery after surgery, injuries, or burns by enhancing tissue regeneration and angiogenesis (the formation of new blood vessels).

- **Nerve Repair:** Used for peripheral neuropathy, sciatica, and nerve regeneration after injury.

- **Muscle Recovery:** Popular among athletes for reducing recovery time after workouts or sports injuries.

- **Skin Rejuvenation:** Red and near-infrared wavelengths stimulate collagen and elastin production, improving tone, texture, and elasticity.

- **Dental & Veterinary Uses:** Assists with gum healing, TMJ pain, and even wound recovery in pets.

Some practitioners integrate cold laser therapy into energy-based modalities such as acupuncture or reflexology, applying the laser to acupoints rather than needles, to stimulate the body's meridians with light instead of pressure or metal.

Scientific Validation

Over 5,000 peer-reviewed studies and numerous meta-analyses have confirmed the therapeutic potential of photobiomodulation. Organizations such as the World Association for Laser Therapy (WALT) have established treatment parameters for dosage, wavelength, and power density. The therapy is FDA cleared for conditions such as chronic neck and joint pain, wound healing, and muscle relaxation.

Researchers continue to explore its benefits for neurodegenerative disorders, traumatic brain injuries, and even cognitive enhancement, areas that show great promise as science deepens its understanding of light's effect on neural tissue.

Contraindications and Safety

Cold laser therapy is considered extremely safe when performed within proper clinical parameters. However, it should be avoided for those with overactive cancerous lesions, directly over the thyroid gland or eyes, and in pregnant women over the abdomen (as a precaution). Also, protective goggles are recommended to prevent accidental eye exposure.

Cold Laser Therapy and Digestive Health: Light for the Gut

It might sound surprising, but gentle light can help heal deep within the body—even the digestive system. Essentially, it works anywhere light can penetrate or where energetic pathways connect. Practitioners have found that shining specific wavelengths of red and near-infrared light over the abdominal area can help calm inflammation, improve circulation, and encourage the body's natural repair mechanisms, making it a valuable tool for those with digestive issues.

When used over the stomach, liver, pancreas, or intestines, the light energy is absorbed by the cells, particularly the mitochondria—which respond by increasing ATP production—the fuel for cellular repair. This extra energy helps reduce inflammation in the intestinal lining and enhances the regeneration of mucosal cells that protect the gut barrier. For people with conditions like irritable bowel syndrome (IBS), Crohn's disease, leaky gut, or post-surgical digestive issues, this can be an effective way to restore balance at the cellular level.

Cold laser therapy can be a gentle yet powerful ally for the digestive system. By calming inflammation in the gut, it helps reduce the release of irritating cytokines that damage the intestinal lining. The light energy also supports tissue repair, encouraging the regeneration of the gut's protective mucosa and speeding recovery from damage caused by antibiotics, toxins, or poor dietary habits. As circulation improves, more oxygen and nutrients flow to the digestive organs, helping them function at their best.

Another remarkable effect of cold laser therapy is its ability to balance the nervous system. By influencing the gut-brain axis, it can help quiet the stress responses that often trigger digestive discomfort, bloating, or irregularity. When applied over the liver area, the therapy may also enhance detoxification by improving bile flow, supporting the body's natural cleansing process.

Practitioners often use cold laser therapy over the abdomen to reduce inflammation, along the vagus nerve pathway in the neck to activate the body's "rest and digest" state, and over the liver and gallbladder meridians to enhance detoxification and digestion. It's frequently combined with other energy-based treatments—such as PEMF therapy, frequency-specific microcurrent, or acupuncture to create a deeper energetic reset. Functional medicine clinics have even reported improved outcomes in patients struggling with SIBO, sluggish digestion, or gut dysbiosis when cold laser therapy is part of a comprehensive healing plan that includes nutrition, probiotics, and stress management.

Although cold laser therapy isn't a magic fix for digestive problems, it can be a powerful *complementary tool* that supports the body's natural ability to heal the gut. By reducing inflammation and improving energy flow, this therapy helps the digestive organs restore balance, function more efficiently, and ultimately bring greater comfort and vitality from the inside out.

Cold Laser Therapy for Anti-Aging: Turning Back Time with Light (Yes, you read that right!)

In the world of modern wellness, one of the most remarkable discoveries is that light itself can heal with a gentle yet powerful treatment that uses specific wavelengths of red and near-infrared light to help the body rejuvenate from within. Unlike the harsh lasers used in surgery or skin resurfacing, cold lasers don't burn or damage tissue. Instead, they stimulate the cells' natural ability to repair, regenerate, and renew.

It all starts deep inside the cell, where the mitochondria, our little energy factories, absorb the light photons and respond by producing more ATP, the body's fundamental energy molecule. Think of it as charging your cellular batteries. With more energy, the cells can perform all their vital functions more efficiently, including collagen production, tissue repair, and detoxification. The result is skin that begins to act, look, and feel younger.

Cold laser therapy has become a favorite tool in anti-aging medicine, dermatology, and holistic wellness because it offers visible results without downtime or discomfort. Over time, the light helps smooth fine lines and wrinkles, improve skin tone and texture, and increase elasticity. The gentle beams also stimulate fibroblast activity, the process that encourages the body to build new collagen and elastin, two of the most important proteins for firm, youthful skin.

But the benefits don't stop at beauty. Cold laser therapy enhances circulation and lymphatic flow, bringing more oxygen and nutrients to the skin while helping clear away toxins. This improved microcirculation can brighten the complexion and reduce puffiness, especially around the eyes.

Because it also reduces inflammation, it helps calm the skin and prevent what researchers now call "inflammaging", the slow, cellular wear and tear caused by chronic inflammation.

Many holistic practitioners pair cold laser treatments with PEMF therapy, red light panels, microcurrent facials, or acupuncture for a truly synergistic rejuvenation experience. It can even be used on the scalp to stimulate hair regrowth by improving blood flow to dormant follicles.

Perhaps the most exciting discovery about cold laser therapy is that it doesn't just work on the skin's surface, it supports the body's overall vitality and longevity. By recharging the mitochondria, it can improve energy, accelerate recovery, and promote a sense of youthful well-being that radiates from the inside out.

Cold laser therapy reminds us that light is more than something we see. it's something that *awakens us*. By bathing the body in these gentle frequencies, we are giving our cells the energetic spark they need to remember how to be vibrant, balanced, and alive again.

A Bridge Between Science and Energy Medicine

What makes cold laser therapy especially fascinating is how it elegantly merges Western scientific precision with Eastern energetic principles. Light, frequency, and energy are universal forces, and here they are being harnessed in a way that both modern medicine and holistic healing can appreciate.

In essence, cold laser therapy is not introducing something foreign into the body; it's providing the right energetic conditions for the body to *remember how to heal itself*. From cellular vitality to systemic rejuvenation, this technology exemplifies how the frontier of wellness is shifting from chemical to energetic and from intervention to illumination.

There are many cold laser products from which to choose. Doctors and physical therapists typically use expensive, machine-driven laser devices focused on pain. There are also several available online for home use, with different levels of intensity. The one I have chosen to work with is the ScalarWave. It combines cold laser technology with scalar waves and programmable hertz frequencies that can support nearly every ailment known to man.

Chapter 32
Sound Therapy

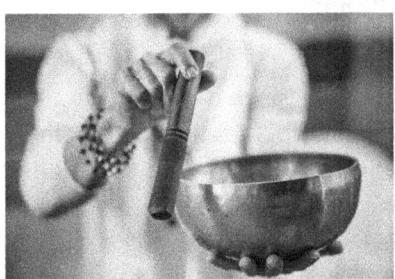

The Healing Power of Sound

The healing power of sound has been recognized since the dawn of time. Ancient civilizations have turned to sound to soothe, energize, and heal. Tibetan monks chant mantras that vibrate through stone walls. Indigenous cultures utilize drum rhythms that echo the heartbeat of the Earth. Ancient Greek physicians prescribed music for melancholy and insomnia. Long before brain scans and frequency analyzers existed, these traditions recognized what modern science now confirms: sound is not merely heard; it is felt, absorbed, and offers profound healing.

How Sound Affects the Body and Mind

Sound is vibration in motion. Every tone, whether from a crystal bowl, ocean wave, or symphony, travels as energy that interacts with the cells, tissues, and subtle energy fields of the body in various ways.

- **Resonance and Entrainment.** Each cell and organ has a natural frequency. When exposed to external vibrations that match or harmonize with that frequency, *resonance* occurs, gently bringing tissues into balance. Rhythmic sound also guides (*entrains*) heart rate, breath, and brainwaves from busy beta activity toward the calm alpha and restorative theta states associated with meditation and deep creativity.

- **Nervous System Regulation.** Low-frequency vibrations stimulate the vagus nerve and activate the parasympathetic "rest-and-digest" system, lowering blood pressure, calming the heart, and reducing stress hormones such as cortisol.

- **Cellular and Molecular Effects.** Research in biophysics suggests that sound influences cellular membranes and may even affect gene expression. In clinical medicine, ultrasound therapy harnesses high-frequency sound to reduce inflammation and accelerate tissue repair.

- **Emotional and Cognitive Healing.** Sound engages many regions of the brain at once, including those governing memory, emotion, and motor control—helping to relieve anxiety and depression, improve mood, and enhance concentration.

Types of Sound Therapy. There are numerous devices and services available that claim to reset your nervous system and offer balance, vitality, and profound inner peace. Some listed below may offer phenomenal healing potential for some and others may not respond favorably to the same modality. If you are new to sound therapy, I invite you to experiment with each one to evaluate their benefits and which ones can be of benefit to you.

Immersive Sound Baths

We have to start with sound bowl therapy because it is my all-time favorite. It is the only therapy I participate in that I always think to myself, "at this moment everything is perfect." Among the many sound-based practices, sound baths are especially transformative. Despite the name, a sound bath is not a bath with water. Instead, it is a *bath of sound waves* that wash over and through the body, saturating every cell in vibration. It's like a spiritual concert for the soul.

Participants typically recline on yoga mats in a softly lit room surrounded by crystal and Himalayan singing bowls, gongs, didgeridoos, chimes, and gentle percussion. The practitioners play these sounds from a stationary spot in the room, and if an instrument is small enough to carry (such as a sound bowl or chimes), it is gently played over each participant.

These sound waves enter the body through the skin, fascia, and bones, where they are felt as subtle pulsations—almost like an internal massage. Many describe sensations of floating, weightlessness, gentle tingling currents, or the spontaneous release of long-held emotions.

Breathing begins to slow, thoughts become quiet, and time seems to dissolve. Some participants report vivid imagery, profound relaxation, or a deep meditative stillness.

Research shows that sound baths can lower heart rate and blood pressure, shift brainwaves from beta to alpha and theta states to promote deep relaxation, creativity, and restorative sleep, reduce cortisol levels, and encourage the release of endorphins and oxytocin, promoting feelings of peace and well-being/ They can also loosen muscular and fascial tension while improving circulation, support emotional processing and a sense of spiritual connection. The result is a full-body reset—participants leave refreshed, centered, and deeply at peace.

Group sessions are quite popular and normally range between $20-$50, depending on the number of practitioners are playing. Private sessions can also be arranged.

Tuning Forks

Tuning forks are used directly on the body or around the energy field. The gentle pulsation can be felt deep within the tissues, like a subtle sonic massage. The sound waves travel through skin, muscle, and bone—stimulating circulation, calming the nervous system, and releasing tension. The body seems to "remember" its own frequency, gradually shifting from chaos to coherence.

Every organ, cell, and atom in the human body vibrates at its own natural frequency. Stress, injury, and emotional strain can throw these frequencies off balance much like an orchestra playing out of tune. Tuning forks act like a conductor's baton, guiding the body back to its original, harmonious vibration.

Studies have shown that sound frequencies can influence brain-wave patterns, slow heart rate, and activate the parasympathetic nervous system—the state where true healing occurs. In clinical settings, vibration therapy has been shown to enhance circulation, relax muscle tension, and promote deep states of calm. While research on tuning forks specifically is still growing, early findings and decades of anecdotal experience point to remarkable benefits for stress reduction, pain relief, and emotional balance.

Tuning forks aren't just for practitioners; anyone can learn to use them with a little guidance and care. The best part is that they are one of the most cost-effective and easy-to-learn tools in the field of sound therapy. Here's what you need to know:

There are two primary kinds of tuning forks used in healing and sound therapy: weighted and unweighted.

- Weighted tuning forks have small metal discs at the ends of each prong. When struck, they produce a gentle, palpable vibration that can be *felt* in the body rather than primarily *heard*. These are typically placed directly on the body—over muscles, joints, bones, acupuncture points, or meridians—to stimulate circulation, release muscle tension, and calm the nervous system. The vibration travels deep into the tissues, much like a subtle form of massage or pulsed energy therapy.

- Unweighted tuning forks have smooth ends and produce a clearer, longer-lasting audible tone. They are used *off the body* for energetic work—sweeping through the aura, balancing chakras, and harmonizing the subtle fields around the body. These are excellent for meditation, emotional clearing, and creating a sense of calm and expansion.

Every tuning fork vibrates at a specific frequency, measured in hertz (Hz), and each frequency has unique properties and effects.

- **128 Hz – The Grounding Fork.** A classic starting point for healing. The 128 Hz weighted fork helps reduce pain, improve circulation, and calm the nervous system. It's also known to encourage the release of nitric oxide—a molecule that supports healthy blood flow and cellular repair.

- **136.10 Hz – The OM Fork.** This tone corresponds to the Earth's annual orbit around the sun and resonates deeply with natural rhythms. When used in meditation or placed near the heart, it brings grounding, relaxation, and a feeling of being aligned with the pulse of the planet.

- **256 Hz and 512 Hz – The Perfect Octave.** These two forks are often used together to create harmonic balance between the left and right hemispheres of the brain. Their pure tones sharpen mental clarity, support focus, and promote equilibrium.

- **528 Hz – The Love Frequency.** Sometimes called the "miracle tone," this fork is associated with the heart chakra, DNA repair, and emotional transformation. It is said to open the heart, uplift the spirit, and restore harmony at a cellular level.

- **4096 Hz – The Angel Fork.** Known for its crystalline clarity, this fork produces a bright, ethereal tone that instantly elevates a room's energy. Used around the head and aura, it is believed to clear stagnant energy and reconnect one's awareness with higher consciousness.

Another group of forks is the Solfeggio scale; an ancient sequence of sacred tones used in Gregorian chants and spiritual music. Each frequency is believed to affect consciousness in specific ways:

- **396 Hz** – Liberates guilt and fear, helping release emotional blockages.

- **417 Hz** – Encourages positive change and clears negativity from past experiences.

- **528 Hz** – Restores harmony, associated with love and cellular repair.

- **639 Hz** – Enhances connection, compassion, and relationship healing.

- **741 Hz** – Supports detoxification, purification, and clear self-expression.

- **852 Hz** – Awakens intuition and higher awareness.

- **963 Hz** – Represents unity, oneness, and connection to universal consciousness.

Though modern science has not fully verified these ancient claims, countless sound healers and wellness practitioners report profound shifts in mood, clarity, and energy when using the Solfeggio tones.

When building your own set, it is recommended to start with a weighted 128 Hz fork for physical work and an unweighted 4096 Hz fork for energy clearing for the perfect foundational pair. As you grow more comfortable, you can expand into chakra sets, Solfeggio sets, or specialized forks that call to you intuitively.

Always strike the fork on a rubber activator—never on metal—and listen for how your body responds. The tones that feel peaceful, expansive, or grounding are your unique resonance. Over time, you'll develop a personal relationship with sound itself, learning to use vibration as both medicine and meditation.

High-quality tuning forks may be purchased through reputable wellness suppliers and sound therapy brands such as BioSonics, Omnivos, Ohm Therapeutics, and Sacred Waves. They're also widely available through Amazon and other online healing boutiques. Look for forks made from heat-treated, medical-grade aluminum alloy for clear, long-lasting resonance. Avoid cheap decorative forks or "toy" sets, as their tuning may not be precise. There are numerous how-to videos on YouTube to teach technique.

The Healing Power of Music

Music is so much more than entertainment. From ancient temples to modern hospitals, music has long been recognized as one of humanity's oldest medicines. Archaeological records show that as far back as 40,000 years ago, early humans crafted flutes from bone for ritual and healing. Ancient Egyptians used chanting to restore harmony to the body; Greek physicians like Pythagoras prescribed specific modes and intervals to balance emotions; and Indigenous cultures across the world used drums, rattles, and songs to restore spiritual and physical health.

Modern science now confirms what our ancestors intuitively knew: sound affects biology. Music can slow the heart rate, lower blood pressure, reduce cortisol, and trigger dopamine and endorphin release. It activates both hemispheres of the brain, harmonizing logic and creativity, and supports neuroplasticity, the brain's ability to rewire and heal.

Every musical note carries a measurable frequency, and each octave doubles the previous frequency. Certain octaves and tunings appear to have stronger biological resonance. For example, 528 Hz—sometimes called the "love frequency"—has been studied for its effects on reducing stress hormones and increasing cellular vitality. Lower octaves, such as gentle drum beats around 60–80 bpm, tend to synchronize with the resting heart rate and promote relaxation, while higher octaves can energize and uplift.

Some music therapists use isochronic tones, binaural beats, or specific harmonic intervals to entrain brainwaves into states of calm (alpha/theta) or focus (beta/gamma). This is the same principle used in meditation and sound baths where the body naturally tunes itself to the dominant vibration in its environment.

In the early 1990s, researchers began studying an intriguing phenomenon now known as the Mozart Effect—the idea that listening to certain classical music, particularly compositions by Wolfgang Amadeus Mozart, can enhance brain function and improve well-being.

The concept first gained attention in 1993, when a study published in the journal *Nature* by Dr. Frances Rauscher, Gordon Shaw, and Katherine Ky showed that college students who listened to Mozart's *Sonata for Two Pianos in D Major (K.448)* for ten minutes scored higher on spatial-temporal reasoning tests compared to those who sat in silence or listened to relaxation instructions. Their IQ boost was temporary—lasting about 10 to 15 minutes—but it sparked enormous interest in how music influences cognition.

Subsequent research has expanded on this idea, revealing that music with harmonic complexity, rhythm, and structure (such as Mozart's) can synchronize neural firing patterns and strengthen connections between brain regions involved in attention, learning, and memory.

Since then, studies have found that the Mozart Effect, or more broadly, music-induced neurostimulation, can calm the nervous system, aid seizure control, support premature infants, and enhance mood and learning. While the Mozart Effect helped popularize the link between music and the mind, newer research shows that the specific composer is less important than the structure and frequency pattern of the music itself. Any music that is harmonically balanced, emotionally uplifting, and free of lyrical distraction can create similar benefits.

Today we have access to sound beds, illustrating the next evolution of sound therapy, from listening to immersive vibrational healing. While most music therapy is experienced through the ears, sound beds invite the entire body to *feel* the vibration. Also known as vibroacoustic therapy beds, these specialized tables or loungers use transducers or speakers embedded beneath the surface to send gentle low-frequency sound waves through the body.

When you lie on a sound bed, you don't just hear the music, you experience it resonating through your muscles, organs, and bones. The sensation is often described as a massage from the inside out. Sound beds operate on the principle that every cell in the body vibrates at its own frequency. When those frequencies become imbalanced through stress, illness, or emotional strain, external vibration can help restore harmony.

Low frequencies (30–120 Hz) penetrate deeply into tissues, relaxing muscles and easing pain; mid-range tones stimulate circulation and lymph flow, and higher harmonics promote mental clarity and emotional release.

The bed converts these frequencies into mechanical vibrations that move through the body's water-rich tissues (our bodies are roughly 70% water), transmitting healing energy efficiently to every cell.

Research into vibroacoustic therapy (VAT) has shown promising results. A 2014 study published in *Music and Medicine* found VAT reduced pain and muscle tension in patients with fibromyalgia and Parkinson's disease. Another study in *Psychology of Music* (2019) reported improvements in mood and sleep quality among participants after a series of vibroacoustic sessions.

This therapy can be found in integrative wellness centers, spas and energy healing studios, and some luxury resorts and retreat centers. Hospitals and integrative clinics now use sound beds for stress reduction, chronic pain, anxiety, insomnia, and PTSD. There are even home versions, from full-size vibroacoustic loungers to compact sound cushions that deliver localized vibration through Bluetooth-controlled frequencies. Sessions typically last 20–60 minutes. The practitioner selects specific frequencies or musical tracks—often in the 40–80 Hz range to entrain relaxation or energy balance. Some combine the sound bed with guided meditation, aromatherapy, or light therapy for a full multisensory experience. Many users describe sensations of warmth, emotional release, or tingling waves of energy as their nervous system shifts from fight-or-flight into deep parasympathetic calm. For those who struggle to meditate or "quiet the mind," sound beds provide a direct sensory pathway to stillness, balance, and coherence.

Binaural Beats for Sound Healing

Binaural beats work by using the brain's natural tendency to synchronize with external rhythmic stimuli—a process known as *brainwave entrainment*. When you listen to two slightly different frequencies in each ear (for example, 200 Hz in the left ear and 210 Hz in the right), your brain doesn't actually hear two separate tones. Instead, it perceives a third "phantom" tone at the difference between the two frequencies — in this case, 10 Hz.

That 10 Hz corresponds to a specific brainwave range (in this example, the **alpha** range), which is associated with calm focus and relaxation. Depending on the difference in frequencies, binaural beats can help guide the brain into states linked with D**elta** (0.5–4 Hz) for deep sleep and healing, **Theta** (4–8 Hz) for meditation, intuition, creativity, **Alpha** (8–12 Hz) for relaxation and mental clarity, and **Beta** (13–30 Hz): alertness and concentration.

By wearing headphones, each ear receives its distinct tone, allowing the brain to generate this internal frequency difference. Over time, this can promote relaxation, focus, or sleep, depending on the frequency used, making binaural beats a popular and accessible form of sound healing.

Numerous soundtracks can be found on YouTube for free. Channels like Good Vibes and Sound Health Solutions provide many choices for various ailments such as headaches, better focus, knee and joint pain, etc., or you can use the search term "binaural beats for (name of ailment)."

Chapter 33
Color Therapy

The Healing Power of Color Therapy

Color therapy, also known as chromotherapy, is based on the principle that color and light can influence our mood, energy, and even physical health. Every color we see corresponds to a specific wavelength of light, each vibrating at its own frequency. Because the human body is essentially an electromagnetic field, it naturally responds to these frequencies.

Ancient civilizations understood this connection long before modern science did. The Egyptians bathed in sun-filled rooms filtered through colored glass; the Greeks used sunlight therapy (heliotherapy) for vitality and balance; and Ayurvedic traditions associated colors with the chakras—energy centers that correspond to the organs and emotions of the body.

Today, color therapy bridges both ancient wisdom and modern research, suggesting that certain wavelengths of light can stimulate biochemical and energetic processes that support healing, mood regulation, and vitality.

How Color Therapy Works

At its core, color therapy operates on the concept of vibrational resonance. Each color carries a specific frequency that can either energize or calm, expand or focus, depending on the body's current state. When a person is exposed to a particular color—through light, visualization, or their surrounding environment—the frequency of that color interacts with the body's own biofield and cellular energy.

From a physiological perspective, light influences hormones and neurotransmitters. For example, exposure to blue light helps regulate circadian rhythms and melatonin production.

Colors affect the autonomic nervous system. Warm tones may elevate heart rate and blood flow, while cool tones can promote relaxation.

On an energetic level, colors are thought to balance the chakras, restoring harmony in areas of the body where energy may be blocked or deficient.

In this way, color therapy doesn't "force" healing; it gently guides the body back to its natural energetic equilibrium—much like tuning a musical instrument back into harmony.

The Color Spectrum and Their Healing Frequencies

Light, though it appears white to the naked eye, is actually made up of a full spectrum of colors—each vibrating at a unique frequency and wavelength measured in nanometers (nm). These wavelengths determine how deeply the light penetrates the body and how it interacts with the cells, nervous system, and energy field. In color therapy, this science meets spirituality: the measurable energy of light aligns with the subtle vibrational energy of the chakras.

Red (620–750 nm)**:** Connects to the root chakra at the base of the spine, red is the longest wavelength and the slowest vibration in the visible spectrum. Because of its penetrating warmth, red stimulates circulation, boosts physical energy, and awakens vitality. It strengthens willpower and helps ground us in the physical body—ideal when we feel tired, fearful, or disconnected. On a cellular level, red light has been used in phototherapy to promote tissue repair and improve blood flow.

Orange (590–620 nm): Resonates with the sacral chakra, orange bridges the grounding qualities of red with the uplifting brightness of yellow. Its frequency stimulates creativity, joy, and sensuality, encouraging emotional release and pleasure in life. Orange light can uplift mood and restore enthusiasm, helping dissolve feelings of guilt or stagnation. Its wavelength gently energizes the reproductive and digestive systems.

Yellow (570–590 nm)**:** Corresponds to the solar plexus chakra, yellow carries a radiant, solar energy that supports confidence, focus, and clarity. This medium wavelength activates the nervous and digestive systems, improving energy metabolism and mood. Yellow encourages optimism and empowerment—it's the color of intellect and personal will. In chromotherapy, it is used to stimulate the mind and dispel fatigue.

Green (495–570 nm): At the center of the spectrum lies green, which aligns with the heart chakra. Its balanced wavelength represents harmony and equilibrium—neither too stimulating nor too calming. Green's frequency nurtures renewal, emotional balance, and physical healing. Scientifically, green light is known to ease migraines and reduce stress responses. Energetically, it opens the heart to compassion and self-acceptance.

Blue (450–495 nm): The Throat Chakra vibrates with the cooling energy of blue. With its shorter wavelength, blue has a calming, anti-inflammatory effect on both body and mind. It soothes stress, reduces blood pressure, and promotes clear communication and self-expression. Blue light therapy is used medically to regulate circadian rhythms and treat certain skin conditions. Spiritually, it helps release fear and encourages speaking one's truth.

Indigo (425–450 nm): Resonates with the Third Eye Chakra, indigo has a deep, introspective vibration that stimulates intuition, insight, and spiritual awareness. Its frequency influences the pineal gland (the "seat of intuition) and supports mental clarity and perception. Indigo light calms overactive thoughts and invites visionary understanding, guiding us toward inner wisdom.

Violet (380–425 nm): The shortest wavelength in the visible spectrum corresponds to the crown chakra. Violet light has the highest frequency, linking it to transformation, spirituality, and higher consciousness. It purifies thoughts, supports meditation, and enhances the connection to the divine. Because of its high vibrational rate, violet helps transmute lower energies into light and awareness.

White Light (Combination of All Wavelengths): Represents Universal Energy. White light encompasses every wavelength of the visible spectrum. It brings harmony and unity, restoring balance across all the chakras. White light therapy is often used for whole-body rejuvenation and emotional purification, symbolizing the merging of physical and spiritual healing.

Receiving Color Therapy with Panels

The ideal way to receiving color therapy is through whole-body emersion through color energy panels. When the body is bathed in color, it's as though each cell remembers its original frequency. Light doesn't just heal—it communicates. These energy panels allow us to reconnect with light as nourishment for both body and soul, reminding us that health is simply harmony in vibration.

At their core, color panels use LED or full-spectrum light technology calibrated to emit precise wavelengths corresponding to specific colors. Each wavelength carries a unique energetic frequency that interacts with both biological tissues and subtle energy systems. The healing light frequencies are absorbed through the skin. When specific wavelengths reach the skin, they penetrate varying depths depending on the color. For example, red light (620–750 nm) penetrates deeply into muscle and connective tissue, stimulating circulation, collagen production, and cellular repair. Blue light (450–495 nm) stays closer to the surface, calming inflammation, supporting skin clarity, and reducing microbial activity. Green and yellow wavelengths influence mood, balance, and overall energy through the nervous system.

A typical color panel session takes place in a tranquil spa or wellness environment. You'll either lie down beneath or between LED panels, or recline inside a light capsule or bed, depending on the setup. Sessions may be accompanied by gentle music or guided relaxation, enhancing the energetic immersion. The duration is normally 20-40 minutes, depending on the color frequencies chosen and individual goals. Some practitioners ask you strip down to the undergarments for better skin exposure. Others ask you to wear white garments, which reflect and distribute light more evenly. After the session, most clients describe sensations of warmth, lightness, and emotional clarity. Others notice improved skin tone, energy levels, and mental focus over time with regular treatments.

Color energy panels are becoming increasingly available and can be found in different types of wellness environments.

- Integrative Wellness Centers & Holistic Spas. Many high-end spas now include chromotherapy rooms or light beds as part of detox or rejuvenation programs.

- Biohacking & Longevity Clinics. Facilities focusing on red light, PEMF, and frequency-based therapies often feature multi-wavelength LED panels for full-spectrum light exposure.

- Energy Medicine Studios & Sound Healing Centers. Some centers combine light with sound frequencies or vibrational beds for a multi-sensory healing experience.

Safety and Frequency of Use

Color energy panel treatments are non-invasive and generally safe for most individuals. However:

Start gradually with 1-2 sessions per week, increasing to 3 as your body adapts.

Hydrate well before and after sessions to support detoxification and energy flow.

Avoid use if pregnant, light-sensitive, or taking photosensitizing medications (consult your practitioner).

Consistency yields the best results; regular exposure helps the body "entrain" to the therapeutic light frequencies.

Receiving Color Therapy Through Glasses

Color therapy glasses are one of the simplest and most enjoyable ways to experience chromotherapy. They are inexpensive and can be purchased on Amazon individually or as a set of each color by searching "color therapy glasses". These specially tinted lenses filter natural or artificial light into a specific color wavelength that gently enters through the eyes and influences the body's energetic and neurological systems.

When light passes through the retina, it stimulates the hypothalamus and pineal gland—regions of the brain that regulate hormones, sleep-wake cycles, mood, and energy balance. Each color lens delivers a different frequency to these centers, subtly shifting biochemical and emotional responses. In essence, the glasses act as portable frequency tuners for the mind and body. The eye doesn't only "see" light—it converts light into neural impulses. When a colored wavelength reaches the retina, it travels via the optic nerve to the hypothalamus, triggering hormonal cascades that influence mood, alertness, and even metabolism.

Emerging research in photobiomodulation suggests that certain wavelengths of visible light may influence mitochondrial energy production. Though color therapy glasses use less intensity than clinical light devices, consistent gentle exposure can still encourage improved vitality, mood, and emotional regulation.

You can choose colors intuitively—trust which tint you feel drawn to—or alternate based on your emotional or physical needs.

Red / Orange: Stimulates energy, confidence, creativity, and circulation. Great for low mood or fatigue.

Yellow: Encourages optimism and focus, helpful for brain fog or lack of motivation.

Green: Balances emotions and relieves tension, ideal for stress or emotional healing.

Blue: Calms the mind and reduces anxiety, useful for overthinking or insomnia.

Indigo / Violet: Supports intuition and meditation; enhances spiritual clarity.

There is no rigid rule, as tolerance and sensitivity vary by individual, but these are generally accepted guidelines:

Start gradually. Begin with 10–15 minutes once or twice a day, ideally in a calm environment or during meditation. I find wearing them outside in natural sunlight feels best. Don't be alarmed if after your session, your color vision is distorted. It will revert back in a few minutes.

Increase slowly — As your system adjusts, sessions can extend to 20–30 minutes or used as needed throughout the day.

For focus or mood support — Wear during work, reading, or creative activities.

For relaxation. Use in the evening with calming tones such as blue or green.

Avoid overexposure. More is not necessarily better. Overuse of stimulating colors (like red or orange) may cause restlessness or eye strain.

The key is consistency and mindfulness. Most users notice subtle mood shifts or energy balancing after several days of use. Color therapy glasses are considered complementary tools, not medical treatments. Those with light sensitivity, migraines, or specific eye conditions should exercise caution and experiment with shorter sessions.

As a sidenote, color therapy works just as effectively for people with color blindness (color vision deficiency). Even when someone cannot *see* a particular color clearly, the wavelength of light still enters the eyes and interacts with the brain and endocrine system. The photoreceptors in the retina (rods and remaining cones) still register light intensity and send electromagnetic information through the optic nerve to the hypothalamus and pineal gland, the same regions influenced in color therapy. So, while a color-blind person may not consciously perceive, say, "vivid red," the biological and energetic response to that wavelength (620–750 nm) can still occur. The body responds to light energy, not just the visual interpretation of color. This is why phototherapy and light-based medical treatments work even for individuals with impaired color vision.

# Chapter 34
Scalar Energy

Scalar energy (sometimes called *scalar waves* or *longitudinal waves*) is a unique form of energy that exists beyond conventional electromagnetic energy, characterized by its non-linear properties and potential applications in holistic health and wellness. It is often referred to as zero-point energy or quantum energy, a concept that originates from the field of quantum physics. Unlike conventional electromagnetic energy, scalar energy is believed to be a non-linear, non-Hertzian form of energy that exists in a different dimensional space. This unique form of energy is thought to have the potential to influence physical matter and biological systems, making it a topic of interest in holistic health practices.

The science behind scalar energy is rooted in the theories of Nikola Tesla and other scientists who explored the nature of energy and its interaction with the universe. Scalar energy is characterized by its ability to exist without a frequency or wavelength, which sets it apart from traditional forms of energy. This energy is often described as a field that permeates the universe, providing a foundation for various natural phenomena and holistic healing practices. These waves of energy are non-Hertzian waves and don't follow the conventional laws of physics because they claim to travel faster than the speed of light and are not diminished by distance. Because science, as it stands, does not have proof that anything moves faster than the speed of light, causes skepticism in the world of science. As such, the power of these mystical claims, allow scalar waves to penetrate various materials and interact with biological systems in profound ways, making them a focal point in holistic health research.

Nonetheless, in the realm of holistic health, scalar energy is believed to promote healing and well-being by restoring balance to the body's energy systems. This type of energy is said to enhance cellular function, improve circulation, and support detoxification processes. By harnessing this energy, individuals may experience increased vitality, reduced stress, and an overall sense of harmony within their bodies.

Scalar energy is utilized in various applications, including wellness devices, therapeutic tools, and energy-enhancing products. Many holistic health practitioners incorporate scalar energy technology into their practices, using devices that emit scalar waves to promote healing. These applications range from scalar energy pendants and mats to advanced therapeutic equipment designed to enhance the body's natural healing processes.

While scalar energy is nothing new (with roots based in 19th-century physics), It has recently become a cultural phenomenon in the holistic arena when EESystems (Energy Enhancement System) started popping up in wellness centers all around the world, one-by-one. It is a unique model where a participant will enter a communal room with several recliners, dim lights, relaxing music and (up to) 48 screens around the room emitting these healing frequencies to be absorbed within an hour or two. It may be worth a try for the experience alone. Some people experience profound healing shifts while others feel nothing more than a relaxing experience and a good nap. Either way, healing frequencies are being absorbed by the body whether it is felt or not.

Chapter 35
The Biomat

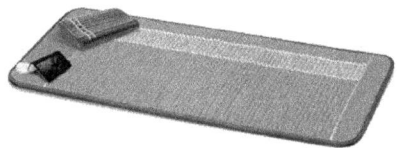

The Biomat: Harnessing Far Infrared and Negative Ions for Deep Healing

The Biomat is a therapeutic mat that merges far infrared light, negative ions, and amethyst crystals to promote relaxation, detoxification, and cellular rejuvenation. Bridging modern biophysics with ancient crystal healing, it delivers deep warmth that nurtures the body's natural ability to restore balance and vitality.

Origins and Development

The Biomat was developed by Richway International, Inc., a South Korean wellness company founded in the late 1990s. The technology was inspired by NASA research on far infrared light, which was found to sustain cellular health in astronauts deprived of natural sunlight. By combining this advanced infrared technology with the energetic amplifying qualities of amethyst quartz, Richway created a portable healing device designed for both clinical and home use.

Today, the Biomat is recognized as an FDA-registered Class II medical device, cleared for temporary relief of muscle pain, joint stiffness, and improved circulation. It's used in holistic clinics, chiropractic offices, and wellness centers worldwide.

How the Biomat Works

Inside the Biomat are layers of amethyst crystals, tourmaline, and natural cotton fibers that work together to convert electricity into far infrared (FIR) rays, gentle, invisible waves of heat that penetrate deep into the body.

Unlike standard heating pads that only warm the surface, far infrared energy heats the body from within, gently raising core temperature, stimulating blood flow, and encouraging the body to release toxins. Simultaneously, the Biomat emits negative ions, the same molecules generated by waterfalls, mountain air, and ocean waves, known for promoting calmness and improved serotonin levels.

The combined effect is a unique synergy of thermal therapy and energetic alignment, warming tissues, relaxing muscles, and helping restore vibrational harmony throughout the body. Far Infrared Rays (FIR) provide wavelengths of 5–15 microns that are absorbed by the body at the cellular level, increasing microcirculation and oxygen delivery to tissues. This helps remove metabolic waste and supports the mitochondria (the cell's power plants) to produce more ATP (energy).

The negative ions bind to free radicals, helping to neutralize oxidative stress. Studies suggest exposure to negative ions may elevate mood, enhance alertness, and even improve sleep quality by balancing serotonin levels. And last but not least, the amethyst crystals act as a natural conductor, amplifying and purifying the FIR waves. Its molecular lattice helps distribute the heat evenly and is believed to carry a subtle, stabilizing frequency that calms the nervous system. Together, these mechanisms enhance circulation, detoxification, and energy coherence, creating a measurable physiological and subtle energetic effect.

Users often describe a Biomat session as "a warm wave of peace." Clinical studies and user experiences highlight a wide range of benefits including:

- **Pain & Inflammation Relief:** Improves circulation and oxygen delivery to ease stiffness and chronic pain.

- **Detoxification:** Encourages sweating and lymph flow to assist the body in removing toxins and heavy metals.

- **Immune Boosting:** The mild increase in core temperature mimics a therapeutic fever response, strengthening immune resilience.

- **Deep Relaxation & Better Sleep:** The release of negative ions calms the nervous system, helping the body enter a parasympathetic "rest-and-digest" state.

- **Anti-Aging & Cellular Renewal:** By enhancing mitochondrial function, FIR energy may help repair damaged cells and slow oxidative aging.

Many practitioners use the Biomat in conjunction with Reiki, massage, PEMF therapy, infrared saunas, or acupuncture, where it amplifies the therapeutic effects of these modalities. However, this therapy can be used as a stand-alone treatment for anyone seeking holistic restoration. It's especially beneficial for those dealing with chronic pain or inflammation (arthritis, fibromyalgia, muscle tension), stress, anxiety, or insomnia, low energy or adrenal fatigue, circulatory issues and poor detoxification, immune challenges or recovery from illness

Safety and Considerations

While the Biomat is safe for most individuals, those who are pregnant, have a pacemaker, or suffer from serious cardiovascular disease should consult their healthcare provider before use. Sessions can range from 20 to 60 minutes, with temperature settings adjusted for comfort and therapeutic goal. Hydration before and after is essential, as the body naturally releases toxins through sweating.

The Biomat represents the next step in energy-based wellness, uniting light, crystals, and natural ionization to help the body remember what it already knows: how to heal itself. When used consistently, it can serve as a daily anchor of warmth, relaxation, and renewal, literally raising your vibration from the inside out.

Chapter 36
Wearable Frequency Patches

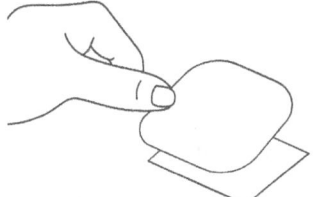

The Future of Healing: Wearable Frequency Patches

Imagine sticking a small, paper-thin patch on your body and feeling calmer, sleeping better, or noticing a boost of energy — all without a single chemical entering your body. It sounds futuristic, yet wearable frequency patches are quietly becoming one of the most intriguing frontiers in holistic wellness and energy medicine.

These little discs of adhesive technology are designed to *communicate* with the body rather than medicate it. They claim to work through light, subtle energy fields, or microcurrents to help the body remember what balance feels like by nudging it back toward its natural state of harmony. Let's dig in to see if they really work or if there's a placebo effect going on.

Frequency Patches vs. Drug-Based Patches

At first glance, a frequency patch may look just like a traditional transdermal patch, but the way it works is completely different. The key difference lies in what each one delivers to the body.

Conventional transdermal patches, such as nicotine, hormone, or pain-relief patches, use a chemical delivery system. They contain active pharmaceutical ingredients that are designed to be absorbed through the skin and into the bloodstream. These patches depend on the movement of molecules through the skin barrier, often assisted by adhesives, heat, or chemical agents that enhance absorption. The purpose is to deliver a specific, measurable dose of a drug or nutrient to create a desired biological effect — for example, to relieve pain, balance hormones, or reduce nicotine cravings. In short, drug-based patches work on a biochemical level.

Frequency patches, by contrast, do not contain any drugs, chemicals, or measurable substances. Instead, they are designed to deliver energy, or more precisely, *information* to the body. These patches are often made from biocompatible materials such as polymer films, silicon layers, or special non-conductive fabrics that can be "imprinted" or "charged" with specific vibrational frequencies. When placed on the skin, the patch interacts with the body's natural electromagnetic field, transmitting subtle energetic signals that help restore balance to cellular communication. Rather than forcing a chemical change, frequency patches are believed to influence the body's biofield, supporting its natural ability to self-regulate and heal.

The difference, therefore, is profound. A drug-based patch works by introducing chemistry into the body, while a frequency patch works by influencing energy. One alters the body's chemistry directly; the other communicates information through resonance. Both approaches share the same goal to promote health and balance but they operate on completely different principles. The emerging field of energy and frequency medicine views the body not merely as a biochemical system but as an energetic matrix that can respond to subtle vibrational cues, much like a musical instrument that retunes itself when it comes into harmony with a new frequency.

How They Work: Light, Signals, and Subtle Energy

Every cell in the human body vibrates and emits tiny electrical and light signals. When we're healthy, these signals are coherent, like a well-tuned orchestra. When stress, toxins, or aging disrupt that harmony, the "music" of the body can fall out of sync.

Frequency patches attempt to re-tune the system by interacting with the body's biofield. They do this in a few different ways:

1. **Phototherapy Patches**

Some patches use the body's own infrared heat to reflect specific wavelengths of light back into the skin. This gentle light (a form of *photobiomodulation*) can signal the cells' energy centers (the mitochondria) to produce more ATP, the body's cellular fuel. In simpler terms: they may help your body recharge its batteries naturally.

This process is similar to what happens during light therapy or red-light treatments, but in a far subtler, wearable form.

2. **Microcurrent and Frequency Stimulation**

Another category delivers soft, electrical pulses, so gentle you don't feel them, to stimulate cellular repair or calm pain signals. These microcurrents are cousins to the ones used in physical therapy and facial rejuvenation devices. The goal is to restore communication between cells, muscles, and nerves.

3. **Imprinted or Nanotech Patches**

Then there's the more mysterious kind: patches "imprinted" with energetic frequencies of natural substances or structured materials that are said to influence the body's energy field through resonance. While the science here is emerging and sometimes debated, many users report noticeable shifts in energy, mood, and pain relief.

Leading Brands and Their Approaches

LifeWave®

Perhaps the most well-known name in the space, LifeWave creates non-transdermal light-reflecting patches such as the X39®, designed to activate the body's natural production of the peptide *GHK-Cu*, linked to repair and regeneration. Other patches target sleep, energy, mood, and detox. Though their studies are small, many users describe improved sleep, focus, and faster recovery, suggesting that subtle light-based signaling may indeed influence biological rhythms. David Schmidt, the found of LifeWave, set the company up as a multi-level distribution marketing format, meaning you need to purchase through an independent distributor. Back in 1999, I tried out the X39 patch for approximately six months and did not notice any difference in energy levels, and if I did, they may have been subtle. Due to the hefty price tag on these, I discontinued its use. This is a prime example of how there is not a one-product-fits-all modality. Some things work great for some, while others may not receive the same results. However, today, many people I personally know continue to use them consistently with favorable testimonials. They are now sold everywhere, including Amazon.

Healy®

Healy takes a slightly different approach. It's a wearable microcurrent device that pairs with adhesive pads and runs specific frequency programs through the body for relaxation, pain relief, or vitality. Think of it as a portable frequency therapist that speaks to your cells in gentle electrical whispers.

Kailo™ and NeuroCuple™

These nanotech patches claim to interact with the body's electrical signals to reduce pain. Users simply place them near the discomfort area, and many report noticeable relief within minutes. Though scientists debate the mechanism, the real-world testimonials are hard to ignore.

LUMINAS®

These patches are "electron-charged" with natural frequencies from minerals and plants. The company describes them as energy batteries that help reduce inflammation and discomfort, without chemicals or side effects.

Frequency Apps

These patches help you conquer whatever ailment you may be facing. From clearing acne to bone and joint health, mental health, boosting your immune system, and more. Their website can be viewed at www.FrequencyApps.com.

What People Are Reporting

Pain Relief: Users frequently report that sore joints, back pain, and muscle aches ease after applying patches — sometimes within minutes.

Better Sleep: Calming frequency blends appear to help regulate circadian rhythms and deepen rest.

Increased Energy: By supporting cellular voltage and circulation, some patches make people feel more alert and vital.

Youthful Glow: Light-based patches are even marketed for skin rejuvenation, collagen support, and improved healing.

Emotional Balance: Because frequencies influence the nervous system, many users feel calmer, more centered, and less reactive.

The Science and the Mystery

Research on wearable frequency patches is still in its early stages. There's solid evidence behind light and microcurrent therapies in general and have been used for decades in sports medicine and wound healing, but much less independent study on specific patch brands. Still, the idea that the body can be *informed* rather than *forced* resonates deeply with the future of energy medicine.

In the holistic model, the body isn't a machine to be fixed; it's an intelligent field of vibration that can be reminded of its own perfection. Frequency patches are tools of remembrance, subtle signals that whisper: *"You already know how to heal."*

Safe and Smart Use

Start slow — try one patch at a time for a few hours. Rotate locations to prevent skin irritation. Drink extra water (electrical flow needs hydration). Don't use over open wounds, near pacemakers, or while pregnant without professional advice. Log your results: note sleep quality, mood, energy, and pain levels for two to four weeks. You may see patterns emerge.

The Bigger Picture

Wearable frequency patches are part of a larger movement toward "information medicine", healing through resonance rather than resistance. Whether they work through light, subtle current, or simply through intention amplified by technology, their growing popularity reflects a deeper truth: *energy is the new frontier of wellness.* I like the idea of receiving healing frequencies in this convenient format. It is my hope that this technology continues to grow with emerging brands, uses, and reasonable pricing.

When combined with clean nutrition, emotional release, movement, meditation, and self-care, these patches can become small allies on your journey to radiant, balanced living, proof that sometimes, the smallest things can make the biggest energetic difference.

Chapter 37
PEMF

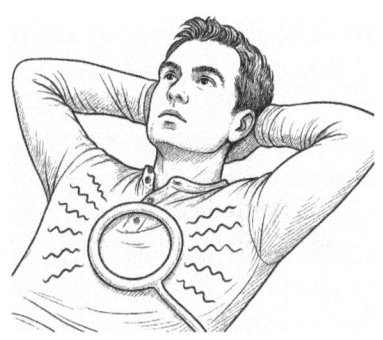

In our modern world, surrounded by artificial frequencies from phones, Wi-Fi, and electronics, it's easy to forget that our bodies are electric by nature. Every heartbeat, every thought, and every cell function depends on subtle electromagnetic communication. Pulsed Electromagnetic Field (PEMF) therapy is designed to restore this natural communication, gently recharging the body at the cellular level and promoting a state of balance and vitality.

What Is Pulsed Electromagnetic Field (PEMF) Therapy?

PEMF therapy uses low-frequency electromagnetic waves that pulse through the body to stimulate cellular repair and enhance natural energy production. These frequencies mimic the Earth's natural electromagnetic field — the same gentle Schumann resonance that our bodies evolved with before modern interference.

A PEMF device typically consists of a mat, pad, or coil that emits these pulses at specific intensities and durations. When the body is exposed to these electromagnetic fields, the energy penetrates deep into tissues, bones, and even individual cells. This re-energizes the mitochondria, the "powerhouses" of the cells, improving oxygenation, circulation, and detoxification while reducing inflammation and pain.

Who Invented PEMF Therapy?

The roots of PEMF therapy trace back to the early 20th century. by non-other than the great pioneer of electromagnetism, Nikola Tesla. He first demonstrated that pulsed magnetic fields could influence the human body's energy and electrical balance. In the 1950s and 1960s, Eastern European and Soviet scientists further developed the technology, using PEMF to help astronauts maintain bone density and muscle strength in zero gravity.

NASA later conducted its own research in the 1990s and early 2000s, confirming that specific electromagnetic frequencies could stimulate the growth and repair of human tissues. Since then, PEMF devices have become widely available for both medical and home use, with FDA clearance for applications such as bone healing, depression, and post-surgical pain.

How PEMF Works: A Cellular Recharge

Our cells maintain an electrical potential across their membranes, a voltage that determines how well nutrients enter and waste exits. When the membrane potential weakens due to stress, toxins, or aging, the cell becomes sluggish. PEMF therapy helps restore this voltage by generating a mild electromagnetic pulse that "charges" the cell, much like plugging in a drained battery.

The result is improved energy production, enhanced repair, and more efficient communication between cells. Over time, this translates to better overall function of the body's systems.

Health Benefits of PEMF Therapy

Scientific and clinical studies have shown that PEMF therapy can:

- Reduce pain and inflammation by modulating inflammatory cytokines and promoting circulation.
- Enhance cellular regeneration and tissue repair.
- Improve sleep and stress resilience by supporting natural mela-

tonin and serotonin cycles.

- Increase energy and vitality through improved mitochondrial performance.
- Accelerate bone healing and recovery after fractures or surgery.
- Support detoxification by improving lymphatic flow and oxygenation.

Many users describe the experience as deeply grounding, restorative, and energizing — a feeling of being "recharged from within."

Who Can Benefit from PEMF Therapy?

Essentially, PEMF therapy is for anyone who wants to optimize their body's energy and self-healing potential. PEMF therapy is often recommended for Individuals with chronic pain, arthritis, or inflammation, those recovering from injuries or surgery, people with fatigue, burnout, or low energy, individuals experiencing poor circulation, sleep issues, athletes looking to enhance recovery and performance, older adults seeking support for bone health and longevity. My very first client to receive PEMF therapy at my center broke her bone while jogging by falling off a curb. She came hobbling in on crutches. On her 4th and final visit, she was practically skipping in with tennis shoes. She informed me that her physician (who referred her in the first place) was in shock over how quickly her bone fused.

Contraindications: When PEMF Should Not Be Used

While PEMF therapy is generally safe and non-invasive, there are situations in which it is not recommended. People who should avoid or seek medical supervision before using PEMF therapy include Pregnant women (safety not established), Individuals with pacemakers or implanted electronic devices, as magnetic fields may interfere with their function, those with epilepsy or seizure disorders, patients who have undergone organ transplants, as immune modulation could pose risks. As with any therapy, it's best to consult a qualified health professional before beginning treatment, especially if you have a chronic condition or are on medications.

Experiencing PEMF Therapy

PEMF sessions can be done in clinics, wellness centers, or at home using portable devices. Most treatments last between 15 to 30 minutes, though therapeutic mats and wearable devices can be used daily for longer periods depending on the program.

During a session, you may feel warmth, tingling, or deep relaxation — subtle signs of your body's natural energy flow reawakening. Over time, users often report improved sleep, pain relief, and an overall sense of restored vitality.

PEMF Therapy and Anti-Aging: Recharging the Cells of Youth

One of the more exciting aspects about PEMF is that it is increasingly being explored for its anti-aging effects, both at the cellular and systemic levels. While PEMF isn't a "fountain of youth," it supports many biological processes that slow down cellular aging, improve vitality, and enhance longevity markers naturally. As we age, our cells lose their natural charge, their ability to efficiently take in nutrients, expel waste, and communicate with one another begins to decline. The body's electrical potential weakens, leading to fatigue, inflammation, slower healing, and the visible signs of aging in the skin, muscles, and overall vitality.

PEMF therapy addresses this decline at its root by recharging the body's cells with low-frequency electromagnetic energy that mimics the Earth's natural field. The result is a gentle yet profound rejuvenation effect that can be felt throughout the body in the following ways:

- **Cellular Regeneration and Mitochondrial Health.** At the core of PEMF's anti-aging potential is its influence on mitochondria, the energy-producing "power plants" within each cell. As we age, mitochondrial output declines, leading to lower ATP (adenosine triphosphate) levels, the body's fundamental energy currency. PEMF therapy has been shown in research to stimulate mitochondrial activity, increasing ATP production, improve cellular metabolism, enabling better repair and renewal, and reduce oxidative stress, one of the main contributors to cellular aging. In other words, by supporting mitochondrial function, PEMF essentially turns back the clock on tired cells, allowing them to function as they did in youth.

- **Improved Circulation and Oxygenation.** One of the most visible aspects of aging is a decline in circulation. Sluggish blood flow means cells receive less oxygen and nutrients, while toxins accumulate. PEMF therapy enhances microcirculation, improving oxygen delivery and waste removal at the cellular level. This leads to healthier, more radiant skin, improved nutrient absorption for repair and collagen production, faster tissue recovery and reduced inflammation. Many users describe a "glow" or a feeling of renewed vitality after regular PEMF sessions as a result of the body literally being re-oxygenated and recharged.

- **Collagen Production and Skin Health.** Collagen is the protein that gives our skin firmness and elasticity, but production naturally declines with age. Studies suggest PEMF stimulation can enhance fibroblast activity, the cells responsible for producing collagen and elastin. Regular use of PEMF facial applicators or mats can promote smoother, firmer skin texture, reduce puffiness and inflammation, and accelerate wound or scar healing. Some med-spas even combine PEMF with red light therapy to maximize collagen renewal, pairing cellular energy with light-induced skin rejuvenation.

- **Hormonal Balance and Anti-Inflammatory Effects.** Chronic inflammation is now recognized as a major driver of aging, often called *inflammaging*. PEMF helps calm this process by down-regulating pro-inflammatory cytokines (like TNF-alpha and IL-6), supporting adrenal and hormonal balance, reducing stress-induced wear on the body. This means fewer inflammatory responses, better sleep, and more stable mood and energy levels, all key elements of aging gracefully.

- **DNA Protection and Cellular Longevity.** Emerging evidence suggests that electromagnetic stimulation can influence telomere activity, the protective caps on chromosomes that shorten as we age. Some studies show that optimizing cellular voltage and reducing oxidative damage may slow telomere shortening, helping preserve genetic stability over time. In other words, PEMF doesn't just make you *feel* younger — it may help your cells *age more slowly* at the molecular level.

- **Restorative Sleep and Stress Reduction.** One of the most overlooked anti-aging benefits of PEMF is its effect on the nervous system. By harmonizing brainwave activity and promoting parasympathetic ("rest-and-repair") dominance, PEMF encourages deep, restorative sleep, when most cellular regeneration occurs. Regular users often report better sleep quality and circadian rhythm balance, reduced anxiety and tension, and a calmer, clearer mental state. Since chronic stress accelerates aging, PEMF's ability to balance the nervous system directly supports emotional and physical longevity.

Aging Gracefully Through Energy Balance

Aging is not simply the passage of time — it's the gradual loss of cellular energy and coherence. PEMF therapy helps restore that coherence, reawakening the natural regenerative intelligence within the body. By supporting mitochondrial function, circulation, collagen, and sleep, it helps create the inner environment where longevity can thrive. In essence, PEMF is not just anti-aging — it's pro-vitality. It reconnects us to the very frequencies that sustain life on Earth. It reminds the body of its original blueprint, vibrant, balanced, and self-healing. By aligning with these natural pulses, we restore not just our energy, but our harmony with the living field that surrounds us all.

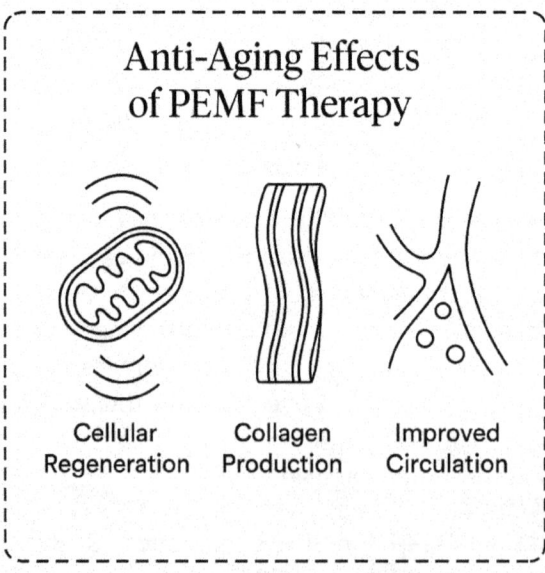

Chapter 38
BioCharger NG

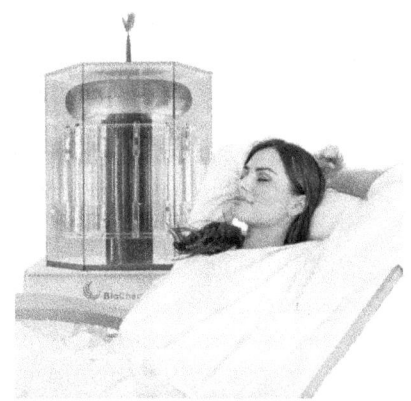

The BioCharger NG, short for *Next Generation*, is a modern wellness device that brings the science of energy medicine into practical use. It's designed to revitalize the body by delivering four types of natural energy simultaneously—light, frequencies, voltage, and pulsed electromagnetic fields (PEMF). Together, these elements are said to re-energize cells, balance the body's biofield, and support overall wellbeing.

The BioCharger draws inspiration from pioneers like Nikola Tesla and Georges Lakhovsky, who believed that energy and frequency form the foundation of health. At its core, this device emits a subtle, non-contact field that surrounds the body. During a session, you simply sit or stand a few feet away while it emits pulsing lights and gentle electromagnetic waves.

Each of the four energies plays a specific role:

- **Light:** Ionized noble gases (such as argon and xenon) create plasma light that interacts with the body's photoreceptors, promoting energy production and repair.

- **Frequencies and Harmonics:** The device transmits a wide range of frequencies that may help the body's cells "tune" back to their optimal resonance.

- **Voltage:** Low-current, high-voltage fields are thought to stimulate the cell membrane and restore electrical balance.

- **PEMF:** Gentle electromagnetic pulses support circulation, oxygenation, and cellular recovery.

The combination of these energy forms mimics the vibrational environment of nature, sunlight, atmospheric energy, and the Earth's magnetic field—all of which are diminished in our modern indoor lifestyles.

The BioCharger NG is pre-programmed with over 1,400 unique "recipes"—carefully developed frequency combinations designed to target specific wellness goals. These recipes cover a wide range of applications, supporting issues such as digestive imbalances, parasites, fatigue, inflammation, viruses, circulation, and stress response. Each session type delivers a distinct energetic pattern intended to harmonize the body's systems and encourage self-repair.

While formal scientific research is still developing, many practitioners and users report noticeable improvements in energy levels, focus, sleep quality, mood, recovery time, and overall sense of wellbeing. The BioCharger is often used as part of an anti-aging or cellular-optimization program and pairs well with other modalities such as red-light therapy, PEMF mats, and infrared saunas.

Sessions are brief—typically fifteen to thirty minutes—and performed while sitting or lounging within a few feet of the device. Most wellness centers or practitioners select specific recipes to match the client's goals, such as vitality, relaxation, immune support, or detoxification. For best results, users are encouraged to hydrate before and after sessions and to approach the experience with calm focus and intention.

The BioCharger NG aligns beautifully with the philosophy of *Radiant Wellness*—that health is an energetic expression of balance and vitality. This technology offers a practical way to recharge the body's electrical potential and restore harmony to the biofield. Used alongside clean nutrition, movement, emotional renewal, and restorative sleep, it becomes part of a holistic system for sustaining energy, longevity, and vibrancy.

Safety and Considerations. The BioCharger NG should not be used for individuals with pacemakers, metal implants, epilepsy, or who are pregnant. Some users experience temporary fatigue or mild detox effects after sessions, which can be balanced with rest and hydration.

About the Author

Denise Cahill is a holistic health practitioner, certified nutritionist, and founder of SoulScans, a groundbreaking biofeedback system that helps identify and clear stored emotional and spiritual blocks, negative patterns, and childhood imprints to promote deep healing and transformation.

With over 25 years of clinical experience in naturopathic health and integrative wellness, Denise combines holistic nutrition with bioenergetic testing—a powerful form of biofeedback that reveals functional disturbances at the cellular level to uncover the root causes of symptoms that traditional testing often cannot identify.

Through her private practice, Denise has guided countless clients toward renewed vitality and emotional well-being by teaching how energy, frequency, and vibration influence both health and consciousness. Her work bridges science and spirituality, helping others restore harmony in body, mind, and soul.

She currently sees clients in her Scottsdale, Arizona office and is developing plans for a wellness resort and retreat center in Playa Flamingo, Costa Rica, dedicated to education, restoration, and radiant living.

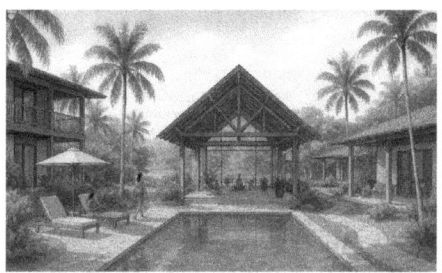

WELLNESS RESORT AND RETREAT CENTER
PLAYA FLAMINGO, COSTA RICA

www.ingramcontent.com/pod-product-compliance
Lightning Source LLC
Chambersburg PA
CBHW060452030426
42337CB00015B/1561